Essential Revision Notes for the FRCS (Urol)

Jack Donati-Bourne

Book 2

First published in 2020 by Libri Publishing

Copyright © Jack Donati-Bourne

The right of Jack Donati-Bourne to be identified as the author of this work has been asserted in accordance with the Copyright, Designs and Patents Act, 1988.

ISBN 978-1-911450-71-9

All rights reserved. No part of this publication may be reproduced, stored in any retrieval system or transmitted in any form or by any means, electronic, mechanical, photocopying, recording or otherwise, without the prior written permission of the copyright holder for which application should be addressed in the first instance to the publishers. No liability shall be attached to the author, the copyright holder or the publishers for loss or damage of any nature suffered as a result of reliance on the reproduction of any of the contents of this publication or any errors or omissions in its contents.

A CIP catalogue record for this book is available from The British Library

Cover and Design by Carnegie Publishing

Libri Publishing
Brunel House
Volunteer Way
Faringdon
Oxfordshire
SN7 7YR

Tel: +44 (0)845 873 3837

www.libripublishing.co.uk

CONTENTS

ACKNOWLEDGEMENTS	V
INTRODUCTION	XI
GLOSSARY OF ABBREVIATIONS	XIII
STATION 5: CALCULI AND URINARY TRACT INFECTIONS	1
STATION 6: UROLOGICAL IMAGING & PRINCIPLES OF UROLOGICAL TECHNOLOGY	97
STATION 7: BLADDER DYSFUNCTION AND GYNAECOLOGICAL ASPECTS OF UROLOGY	159
STATION 8: BPH AND ANDROLOGY	221
ANSWERS TO MCQS	301
STATION 5: CALCULI AND URINARY TRACT INFECTIONS	301
STATION 6: UROLOGICAL IMAGING & PRINCIPLES OF UROLOGICAL TECHNOLOGY	302
STATION 7: BLADDER DYSFUNCTION AND GYNAECOLOGICAL ASPECTS OF UROLOGY	302
STATION 8: ANDROLOGY AND BPH	303

ACKNOWLEDGEMENTS

Taking on and passing the FRCS (Urol) is a team effort – I would never have managed on my own.

I wish to thank my "triple-A" rated revision group – Anthony (Noah), Adeel (Khan) and Ahmed (Kodera). They taught, supported and accompanied me throughout the long journey to the end, I hope I was able to help you as much as you all helped me – indeed we still have our FRCS (Urol) WhatsApp group to this day.

Many colleagues kindly gifted their precious time to help with exam advice and viva practice, I hope I have included all of them. Thank you to Rupesh Bhatt, Anand Dhanasekaran, Herman Fernando, David Muthuveloe, Praveen Pillai, Philip Polson, Hosam Serag, William Taylor, Rebecca Tregunna and Dan Wood.

Finally, I am very grateful to the authors of "Viva Practice for the FRCS (Urol) and Postgraduate Urology Examinations" (Arya M et al.) – your book was of great assistance and was the only light I had to guide me through the exam darkness. I hope my book will now complement yours and together we can support FRCS (Urol) candidates in the future.

For the production of this book I wish to thank Roger Amos, Celia Cozens and John Sivak from Libri Publishing for having faith in me and my project at the beginning and providing fantastic support throughout the publication process.

For support during particularly difficult exam times I am indebted to Harry, Darryl, Suleiman, Jessica, Juan and Aunty Shanaz.

I dedicate this book to my dad – I hope he would have been proud of me if he could read it, to my mum – to whom I owe simply everything, and to Shamah – thank you for teaching me about what really matters in life, I love you.

INTRODUCTION

Thank you for choosing my book!

I do sincerely hope you will find it useful and that above all it helps you pass the FRCS (Urol) exam, which is an important milestone in your career as a urologist and, for many, the last exam in a long series of assessments dating back from medical school.

When preparing for the FRCS (Urol) I often felt that I did not have a clear compass for my revision. Resources for the exam were very scarce, and I was never entirely sure that I was focusing my time and efforts in the right direction. The FRCS (Urol) is stressful enough as it is, and I wanted to take that stress of the "unknown" away for you – and that was the impetus to write this book. I believe that if you read this book in full and use it alongside your other resources, it will serve as a really helpful guide for your revision.

I thought I would briefly share a few of my own reflections with you, mainly to provide encouragement and reassurance that you are not alone if you are feeling stressed, tired and nervous about this exam.

The FRCS (Urol) exam is a tough challenge – it is a taxing exam in itself, but also the time when most take it naturally tends to coincide with a phase in life which for many of us is very busy. Many of you may be newly married or moving in with your partners, expecting or looking after young children, buying a new home… not to mention working a busy hospital job, learning how to operate on patients and who knows maybe even trying to maintain a semblance of a social life!

Furthermore like any skill in life, taking exams is easier with practice and now that you have decided to sit the FRCS (Urol) you may find it has been many years since you last sat down and took time out of your life to prepare for an exam.

Personally I found this to be the biggest challenge of the FRCS (Urol), and whilst there are many things in life we cannot change or control, there are some pieces of advice which I believe are helpful.

Firstly, plan ahead and chose the right moment to take the FRCS (Urol). I strongly recommend you fully focus on the aim to pass both parts first time, but in so doing you have to accept that 6 to 7 months of your life have to be set aside to take the exam and are effectively a write-off. Time the exam such that if possible, you avoid juggling other important commitments such as moving house, having babies or planning weddings. You are much better off nailing the exam first time rather than giving it less than 100% effort and finding yourself having to repeat a station, with all the added stress this entails and the prolonged time with the FRCS (Urol) hanging over your (and your family's) head.

Secondly, do not try to tackle this exam on your own. Speak to senior colleagues who have recently taken the exam (you will find there is always a folder full of exam material saved on somebody's hard drive going round). Form positive connections and revision groups with peers taking the exam with you – group revision is absolutely essential, particularly for the viva. You will not succeed in the viva if you do not practice regularly in your group.

Ensure your family is well aware of the upcoming challenge and that you need their support during this stressful time. Remember we are stronger together.

Lastly, do not worry. The exam is not easy, but it is fair! If you set aside plenty of time, put the right amount of effort and use the correct resources, you will pass. And even if you don't – well, there are many consultants who had to retake it and they are just fine and very successful now!

There are positives – although I had many late nights, tired mornings and missed social events, what I can say is that for probably the first time in my life I found the revision enjoyable. I realised that all the knowledge was directly relevant to my future practice as a urologist. I was finally understanding the rationale and evidence behind my daily clinical practice rather than relying on transcended knowledge from a more senior colleague telling me "this is how it should be done". Finally, when I came out the other end of the FRCS (Urol), I felt so much more confident in hospital and in looking after my patients, which is a priceless and enduring satisfaction to have.

I do wish you all the best with the FRCS (Urol). Good luck!

Jack Donati-Bourne (2020)

GLOSSARY OF ABBREVIATIONS

AAST – American Association for the Surgery of Trauma
AC – assisted conception
ACT – α1 anti-chymotrypsin
ACTH – adreno-corticotropic hormone
AD – autonomic dysreflexia
ADH – anti-diuretic hormone
ADT – androgen deprivation therapy
AFP – alpha feto-protein
AKI – acute kidney injury
ADPKD – autosomal dominant polycystic kidney disease
ALP – alkaline phosphatase
ALPP – abdominal leak point pressure
AMG – α2 macro globulin
AML – angiomyolipoma
ANP – atrial natriuretic peptide
AP – antero-posterior
APD – antero-posterior diameter
APC – adenomatous polyposis coli
ARCD – acquired renal cystic disease
ARR – absolute risk reduction
ASAP – atypical small acinar proliferation
AS – active surveillance
AUA – American Urology Association
AUR – acute urinary retention
AUS – artificial urinary sphincter
BAPU – British Association of Paediatric Urologists
BCI – bladder contractility index
BMD – bone mineral density
BOO – bladder outlet obstruction
BOOI – bladder outlet obstruction index
BPE – benign prostatic enlargement
BPH – benign prostatic hyperplasia
BPS – bladder pain syndrome
BTB – blood-testis barrier
BTx – brachytherapy
BXO – balanitis xerotica obliterans
CAH – congenital adrenal hyperplasia
CAIS – Complete Androgen Insensitivity Syndrome

CAP – continuous antibiotic prophylaxis
CBAVD – congenital bilateral absence of vas deferens
CCG – clinical commissioning group
CCI – Charlson comorbidity index
cCMP – cyclic guanosine monophosphate
CF – cystic fibrosis
CFU – colony forming units
CI – confidence interval
CIS – carcinoma in-situ
CKD – chronic kidney disease
CMV – cytomegalovirus
CN – cytoreductive nephrectomy
CNS – central nervous system
COPD – chronic obstructive pulmonary disease
CPPS – chronic pelvic pain syndrome
CRP – C-reactive protein
CRPC – castrate resistant prostate cancer
CSS – cancer specific survival
CT – computed tomography
CT TAP – computed tomography of thorax abdomen and pelvis
CTU – computed tomography urogram
CVA – cerebrovascular accident
CXR – chest x-ray
DCE – dynamic contrast enhanced
DetSD – detrusor sphincter dyssynergia
DEXA – dual energy absorptiometry scan
DHT – dihydrotestosterone
DLPP – detrusor leak point pressure
DMSA – dimercaptosuccinic acid
DNA – deoxyribonucleic acid
DO – detrusor overactivity
DRE – digital rectal examination
DSD – disorder of sexual differentiation
DSNB – dynamic sentinel node biopsy
DW-MRI – diffusion-weighted magnetic resonance imaging
EAU – European Association of Urology
EBRT – external beam radiotherapy
ECG – electro-cardiogram
ECOG – Eastern Cooperative Oncology Group
ED – erectile dysfunction
EDTA – ethylene diamine tetra acetic acid

EMA – European Medicines Agency
EMRT – emergency medical response team
EORTC – European Organisation for Research and Treatment of Cancer
EPLND – extended pelvic lymph node dissection
EPN – emphysematous pyelonephritis
EPO – erythropoietin
EPR – extra-peritoneal rupture
ERSPC – European Randomised Study of Screening for Prostate Cancer
ESRF – end-stage renal failure
ESWL – extra-corporeal shockwave lithotripsy
ETS – E26 Transformation Specific
FBC – full blood count
FDG – fluorodeoxyglucose
FNA – fine-needle aspiration
FSH – follicle stimulating hormone
FUD – female urethral diverticulum
FVC – frequency volume chart
f/T PSA – free to total prostate specific antigen
GA – general anaesthesia
GAG – glycosaminoglycans
GCNIS – germ cell neoplasia in situ
GCS – Glasgow coma scale
GCT – germ cell tumour
GFR – glomerular filtration rate
GnRH – gonadotropin-releasing hormone
GS – Gram stain
GUCG – Genito-Urinary Cancer Group
HDL – high-density lipoprotein
HEPA – high efficiency particulate air
HGPIN – high grade prostatic intra-epithelial neoplasia
HIFU – high-intensity focused ultrasound
HIV – human immunodeficiency virus
HK – human kallikrein
HLRCC – hereditary leiomyomatosis and renal cell carcinoma
HOLEP – holmium LASER enucleation of the prostate
HPCRU – high pressure chronic retention of urine
HPF – high-powered field
HPG – hypothalamo-pituitary-gonadal
HPRC – hereditary papillary renal cell carcinoma
HPV – human papilloma virus
HU – Hounsfield unit

ICCS – International Children's Continence Society
ICD – implantable cardioverter defibrillator
ICIQ-UI – International Consultation on Incontinence Questionnaire
ICS – International Continence Society
ICSI – intra-cytoplasmic sperm injection
IDO – idiopathic detrusor overactivity
IGF – insulin growth factor
IHD – ischaemic heart disease
IHT – intermittent hormone therapy
IM – intra-muscular
INR – international normalised ratio
IPR – intra-peritoneal rupture
IPSS – International Prostate Symptom Score
ISC – intermittent self catheterisation
ISD – intermittent self dilatation
ISUP – International Society of Urological Pathology
ITGCN – intra-tubular germ cell neoplasia
ITU – intensive therapy unit
IUI – intra-uterine insemination
IV – intra-venous
IVF – in-vitro fertilisation
KSS – kidney sparing surgery
kD – kilo Dalton
LASER – Light Amplification by Stimulated Emission of Radiation
LDL – low-density lipoprotein
LFT – liver function tests
LH – luteinising hormone
LHRH – luteinising hormone releasing hormone
LLN – lower limit of normal
LN – lymph node
LND – lymph node dissection
LPS – lower pole stone
LTC – long term catheter
LUT – lower urinary tract
LUTD – lower urinary tract dysfunction
LUTS – lower urinary tract symptoms
LVI – lymphovascular invasion
MAB – maximum androgen blockade
MAG3 – mercapto acetyltriglycine
MAP – mean arterial pressure
MCDK – multi-cystic dysplastic kidney

mCRPC – metastatic castrate resistant prostate cancer
MCUG – micturating cysto-urethrogram
MDP – methylene diphosphonate
MDRD – Modification of Diet in Renal Disease study
MDT – multi-disciplinary team
MET – medical expulsive therapy
MHRA – Medicines and Healthcare products Regulatory Agency
MHz – mega Hertz
MIBG – metaiodobenzylguanidine
MIS – Mullerian inhibiting substance
mPCa – metastatic prostate cancer
MRU – magnetic resonance (MR) urogram
MV – mega voltage
mL – millilitre
MNE – monosymptomatic nocturnal enuresis
mpMRI – multi-parametric magnetic resonance imaging
mRCC – metastatic renal cell carcinoma
MRI – magnetic resonance imaging
MS – multiple sclerosis
MSU – mid-stream urine (culture)
MUI – mixed urinary incontinence
NA – noradrenaline
NAAT – nucleic acid amplification test
NC – neoadjuvant chemotherapy
NCCT – non-contrast computed tomography
Nd – neodymium
NDO – neurogenic detrusor overactivity
ng – nanogram
NHS – National Health Service
NICE – National Institute of Clinical Excellence
NIDDK – National Institute of Diabetes, Digestive and Kidney Diseases
NNT – number needed to treat
NO – nitric oxide
NPV – negative predictive value
NS – nerve sparing
NSAID – non-steroidal anti-inflammatory drug
NSGCT – non-seminomatous germ cell tumour
NVH – non-visible haematuria
OAB – overactive bladder
OD – once daily
OS – overall survival

PAE – prostate artery embolization
PCa – prostate cancer
PCNL – percutaneous nephrolithotomy
PDD – photo dynamic diagnosis
PDE5i – phosphodiesterase-5 inhibitor
PDGF – platelet-derived growth factor
PET – positron emission tomography
PID – pelvic inflammatory disease
PIRADS – Prostate Imaging Reporting and Data System
PFE – pelvic floor exercises
PFMT – pelvic floor muscle training
PFS – progression free survival
PFUDD – pelvic fracture posterior urethral distraction defect
PN – partial nephrectomy
PO – per oral
POP – pelvic organ prolapse
PPS – prostate pain syndrome
PPV – patent processus vaginalis
PR – per rectum
PSA – prostate specific antigen
PSAD – prostate specific antigen density
PSADT – prostate specific antigen doubling time
PSATZD – prostate specific antigen transitional zone density
PSAV – prostate specific antigen velocity
PSMA – prostate specific membrane antigen
PTFE – polytetrafluoroethane
PTH – parathyroid hormone
PTNS – posterior tibial nerve stimulation
PUJ – pelviureteric junction
PUJO – pelviureteric junction obstruction
PUNLMP – papillary urothelial neoplasm of low malignant potential
PUV – posterior urethral valves
PVD – peripheral vascular disease
PVR – post-void residual
QDS – quarter die sumendum (four times daily)
QOL – quality of life
qSOFA – quick sepsis-related organ failure assessment
RCC – renal cell carcinoma
RCT – randomised controlled trial
RFA – radiofrequency ablation
RN – radical nephrectomy

RNA – ribonucleic acid
RNU – radical nephroureterectomy
RP – radical prostatectomy
RR – relative risk
RTA – renal tubular acidosis
RTB – renal tumour biopsy
RTC – road traffic collision
RTx – radiotherapy
RU – retrograde urethrogram
rUTI – recurrent urinary tract infection
SCC – spinal cord compression
SCCa – squamous cell carcinoma
SCI – spinal cord injury
SFR – stone-free rate
SNM – sacral neuromodulation
SOFA – sequential organ failure assessment
SPC – suprapubic catheter
SPECT – single-photon emission computed tomography
sPSA – super-sensitive prostate specific antigen
SSRI – selective serotonin reuptake inhibitor
STI – sexually transmitted infection
SUI – stress urinary incontinence
TB – tuberculosis
TC – testicular cancer
Tc – technetium
TCC – transitional cell carcinoma
TDS – ter die sumendum (three times daily)
TENS – trans-cutaneous electrical nerve stimulation
TESE – testicular sperm extraction
TIN – testicular intra-epithelial neoplasia
TMPRSS2 – trans-membrane protease serine 2
TOT – trans-obturator tape
TPN – total parenteral nutrition
TRUS – trans-rectal ultrasound
TSG – tumour suppressor gene
TUIP – trans-urethral incision of prostate
TURBT – trans-urethral resection of bladder tumour
TURED – trans-urethral resection of ejaculatory ducts
TURP – trans-urethral resection of prostate
TVT – trans-vaginal tape
UDS – urodynamics

UDT – undescended testis
UE – urea and electrolytes
ULN – upper limit of normal
URS – ureteroscopy
US – ultrasound
USA – United States of America
UTUC – upper tract urothelial cancer
UUI – urge urinary incontinence
VEGF – vascular endothelial growth factor
VH – visible haematuria
VHL – Von-Hippel Lindau syndrome
VIP – vaso-active intestinal peptide
VLPP – Valsalva leak point pressure
VTE – venous thrombo-embolism
VUDS – video urodynamics
VUR – vesico-ureteric reflux
VVF – vesicovaginal fistula
WHO – World Health Organisation
WLE – wide local excision
WW – watchful waiting
XGP – xanthogranulomatous pyelonephritis
YAG – yttrium aluminium garnet
ZA – zoledronic acid
5AR – 5-alpha reductase
5ARIs – 5-alpha reductase inhibitors
5-FU – 5-fluorouracil

STATION 5
CALCULI AND URINARY TRACT INFECTIONS

STONES: BROAD PRINCIPLES

STONE TREATMENTS OVERVIEW

LOWER POLE CALCULI

URETERIC CALCULI

STAGHORN CALCULI

STONES IN SPECIFIC GROUPS

URINARY TRACT INFECTIONS: BROAD PRINCIPLES

RECURRENT URINARY TRACT INFECTIONS

EPIDIDYMO-ORCHITIS

FOURNIER'S GANGRENE

PROSTATITIS

KIDNEY INFECTIONS

CHRONIC PELVIC PAIN

URETHRITIS

URINARY TRACT INFECTIONS IN PREGNANCY

URINARY SCHISTOSOMIASIS

URINARY TUBERCULOSIS

CONTENTS

STONES: BROAD PRINCIPLES — 9
- EPIDEMIOLOGY — 9
- RISK FACTORS — 9
- CLASSIFICATION — 10
  - STONE COMPOSITION — 10
  - RADIO-DENSITY ON X-RAY — 10
  - STONE SIZE / LOCATION — 11
- STONE FORMATION — 11
  - INHIBITORS OF CRYSTALLISATION — 12
- DIFFERENT STONE COMPOSITIONS — 13
  - CALCIUM OXALATE STONES — 13
  - URIC ACID STONES — 14
  - STRUVITE STONES — 16
- IMAGING — 16
  - USS URINARY TRACT — 16
  - NON-CONTRAST CT KUB (NCCT) — 16
  - XR KUB — 18
  - MR UROGRAM — 18
- METABOLIC EVALUATION — 18
- PAIN RELIEF — 19
- RETROGRADE STENT VS. NEPHROSTOMY — 20

STONE TREATMENTS OVERVIEW — 22
- STONE OBSERVATION — 22
- CHEMOLYSIS — 23
- MEDICAL EXPULSIVE THERAPY — 23
- EXTRA-CORPOREAL SHOCKWAVE LITHOTRIPSY (ESWL) — 24
- URETEROSCOPY — 26
- PERCUTANEOUS NEPHROLITHOTOMY — 27

LOWER POLE CALCULI — 30
- BROAD PRINCIPLES — 30
- MANAGEMENT — 30

COMPARING TREATMENTS	31
URETERIC CALCULI	**32**
DIAGNOSTIC EVALUATION	32
MANAGEMENT	32
PHYSIOLOGY OF UPPER TRACT OBSTRUCTION	33
STAGHORN CALCULI	**35**
EPIDEMIOLOGY	35
PATHOLOGY	35
DIAGNOSTIC EVALUATION	36
MANAGEMENT	36
STONES IN SPECIFIC GROUPS	**38**
STONES IN PREGNANCY	38
EPIDEMIOLOGY	38
PATHOPHYSIOLOGY	38
DIAGNOSTIC EVALUATION	39
MANAGEMENT	39
STONES IN CHILDREN	40
STONES IN TRANSPLANT KIDNEYS	41
STONES IN CYSTINURIA PATIENTS	42
EPIDEMIOLOGY	42
PATHOPHYSIOLOGY	42
DIAGNOSTIC EVALUATION	43
MANAGEMENT	43
STONES IN HORSESHOE KIDNEYS	43
MANAGEMENT	44
STONES IN CALCYCEAL DIVERTICULAE	44
STONES IN RENAL TUBULAR ACIDOSIS	45
URINARY TRACT INFECTIONS: BROAD PRINCIPLES	**46**
TERMINOLOGY	46
URINANALYSIS	47
GENERAL APPEARANCE	47
URINE DIPSTICK TEST	47
MID-STREAM URINE CULTURE	49

GRAM STAINING	50
BACTERIAL VIRULENCE VS. HOST DEFENCE	50
ANTIBIOTICS	51
RECURRENT URINARY TRACT INFECTIONS	**53**
DEFINITIONS	53
RISK FACTORS	53
DIAGNOSTIC EVALUATION	54
MANAGEMENT	54
PREVENTION	55
ANTIBIOTIC PROPHYLAXIS	56
SELF-TREATMENT	56
EPIDIDYMO-ORCHITIS	**57**
PATHOGENESIS	57
DIAGNOSTIC EVALUATION	57
MANAGEMENT	58
ORCHITIS	59
FOURNIER'S GANGRENE	**60**
PATHOPHYSIOLOGY	60
DIAGNOSTIC EVALUATION	60
MANAGEMENT	61
PROSTATITIS	**63**
EPIDEMIOLOGY	63
RISK FACTORS	63
DIAGNOSTIC EVALUATION	63
MEARES AND STAMEY TEST	64
MANAGEMENT	65
CHRONIC BACTERIAL PROSTATITIS	65
MANAGEMENT	66
KIDNEY INFECTIONS	**67**
DEFINITIONS	67
ACUTE PYELONEPHRITIS	67
EPIDEMIOLOGY	67

PATHOGENESIS	67
DIAGNOSTIC EVALUATION	68
IMAGING	68
FOLLOW-UP	69
PYONEPHROSIS	69
DIAGNOSTIC EVALUATION	69
IMAGING	69
MANAGEMENT	69
PERI-NEPHRIC ABSCESS	70
DIAGNOSTIC EVALUATION	70
IMAGING	70
MANAGEMENT	70
EMPHYSEMATOUS PYELONEPHRITIS	71
DIAGNOSTIC EVALUATION	71
IMAGING	71
MANAGEMENT	71
XANTHOGRANULOMATOUS PYELONEPHRITIS	72
PATHOLOGY	72
DIAGNOSTIC EVALUATION	72
IMAGING	73
CHRONIC PELVIC PAIN	**74**
DIAGNOSTIC EVALUATION	74
PROSTATE PAIN SYNDROME	75
TREATMENT	75
BLADDER PAIN SYNDROME	76
CLASSIFICATION	76
MANAGEMENT	76
URETHRITIS	**77**
DIAGNOSTIC EVALUATION	77
MANAGEMENT	78
FOLLOW-UP	78
URINARY TRACT INFECTIONS IN PREGNANCY	**79**
EPIDEMIOLOGY	79

MANAGEMENT	79
URINARY SCHISTOSOMIASIS	**80**
EPIDEMIOLOGY	80
PATHOPHYSIOLOGY	80
DIAGNOSTIC EVALUATION	81
TREATMENT	82
SEQUALAE	82
URINARY TUBERCULOSIS	**83**
EPIDEMIOLOGY	83
PATHOGENESIS	83
DIAGNOSTIC EVALUATION	84
URINE CULTURE	84
IMAGING	85
CYSTOSCOPY	85
EFFECTS ON GENITO-URINARY TRACT	85
MANAGEMENT	86
CALCULI AND URINARY TRACT INFECTIONS MCQS	**87**
REFERENCES	**93**

STONES: BROAD PRINCIPLES

EPIDEMIOLOGY

Lifetime risk in developed countries is approximately 10% (men) and 7% (women).

Prevalence of stones is increasing in all Western societies.

Within 1 year of calcium oxalate stone, 10% men will form another, 50% form another in lifetime (further episodes increase recurrence chance and reduces interval between relapses).

Age 20–50 years is the peak incidence for stone formation.

White ethnicity has the highest prevalence of stone disease.

RISK FACTORS

Intrinsic Factors:

- *gender*, men higher risk (testosterone increases oxalate production in liver) (women have higher urinary citrate concentration which inhibits calcium oxalate stone formation)
- *genetic*, more common in Caucasians > Asians > Afro-Caribbean
- *diseases*, including hyperparathyroidism, polycystic kidney disease, Crohn's and Mal-absorption pathologies, obesity / bariatric surgery, gout
- *neurological*, such as MS, spinal cord injury, (bone demineralisation) neurogenic bladder
- anatomy, increased risk with PUJO and horse-shoe kidney
- *UTIs*, due to urease-producing bacteria (proteus, klebsiella, enterobacter)
- *drugs*, corticosteroids (increased gut calcium absorption), chemotherapy [1]

Extrinsic Factors:

- *geographical*, Europe / Scandinavia at higher risk
- *seasonal*, more common in hotter months (peak is one month after summer)

- *dietary*, including high salt and protein intake, low water intake, low calcium intake

CLASSIFICATION

There are many different ways of classifying stones.

These include according to composition, x-ray appearance, size, location, risk of recurrence, aetiology of formation, infection vs. non-infectious causes.

STONE COMPOSITION

The most common stones are made of calcium oxalate – a summary of the different types of urinary tract stones is shown in (Table 2).

80% of uric acid stones are pure, 20% contain calcium oxalate.

The proteinaceous portion of stones is composed of matrix (depending on stone type, kidney stones contain 2.5–65% of non-crystalline matrix).

Table 2 – Summary of different composition of urinary tract stones

Stone Composition	% of all stones
Calcium oxalate	80
Uric acid	10
Calcium phosphate + oxalate	10
Struvite (infection / triple phosphate stones)	10
Cystine	1
Pure calcium phosphate	Rare
Indinavir, triamterene, xanthine	Rare

RADIO-DENSITY ON X-RAY

Three broad categories of stones are described based on their x-ray appearance (Table 3).

Can provide some indication on stone composition and thus determine treatment options.

Table 3 – Categories of urinary tract stones based on their x-ray appearance

X-ray Appearance	Composition
Radio-opaque	Calcium oxalate, calcium phosphate
Poor radio-opacity	cystine, magnesium ammonium phosphate (struvite)
Radio-lucent	Uric acid, drug stones (not visible on CT KUB)

STONE SIZE / LOCATION

Size of stone is usually given in 1–2 dimensions, and stratified as follows:

- < 5mm, 5–10mm, 10–20mm, > 20mm in diameter

Stones can be classified according to anatomical position:

- upper / middle / lower calyx of kidney, renal pelvis, upper / mid- / lower ureter, bladder

Prostatic calculi are usually asymptomatic, they do not affect PSA readings and are made of calcium phosphate / carbonate. [2]

Urethral stones in women are rare and often associated with urethral diverticulum.

STONE FORMATION

Solubility product (K_{sp}) refers to point of saturation where dissolved and crystalline components in solution are in equilibrium.

Driving force behind stone formation is the super-saturation (SS) of urine.

SS occurs when product of concentrations of salts exceeds K_{sp}.

SS is expressed as ratio of urinary calcium oxalate (for example) to solubility, where SS < 1 implies crystals remain soluble, SS > 1 crystals will nucleate and grow.

Above K_{sp} crystals still do not form spontaneously due to inhibitors of formation (although crystallisation can occur on top of pre-existing crystals).

This condition is called the *metastable state*.

However above a certain concentration of salts the inhibitors no longer function and crystals start forming spontaneously.

The concentration above which this process begins to happen is formation product (K_f). [3]

The urine with concentration between K_{sp} and K_f is defined as *metastable*.

Summary of principles using calcium oxalate as an example:
- calcium + oxalate concentration < K_{sp} = no stone formation
- metastable calcium + oxalate concentration = no stone formation
- calcium + oxalate concentration > K_f = stone formation

The process by which nuclei form in pure solutions is called *homogenous nucleation*.

The state of saturation of the urine (saturation index) with respect to particular stone-forming salts indicates the stone-forming propensity of the urine.

Epitaxy

Deposition of one type of crystal upon the surface of another crystal of different composition but similar lattice structure is known as epitaxy.

e.g. uric acid crystals may promote formation of calcium oxalate stones (however rarely cystine)

Randall's Plaques

Although urine is not usually supersaturated with calcium, this may occur in the loop of Henle, leading to precipitation of calcium phosphate in interstitial sites in the inner medulla.

These deposits may develop to the extent that they become visible – these are Randall's plaques.

These plaques have been proposed to act as nidus for development of calcium oxalate stones. [4]

INHIBITORS OF CRYSTALLISATION

Citrate is the only inhibitor of stone formation that is open to manipulation.

Citrate forms soluble complex with calcium, preventing it combining with oxalate / phosphate to agglomerate into crystals.

Citrate therefore lowers the urinary saturation of calcium oxalate.

Primary determinant of urinary citrate excretion is acid-base status (metabolic acidosis reduces citrate excretion as it is metabolised to bicarbonate, alkalosis increases excretion).

Other inhibitors include Tamm-Horsfall proteins, magnesium, glycosaminoglycans.

DIFFERENT STONE COMPOSITIONS

CALCIUM OXALATE STONES

Most patients with calcium oxalate stones have ≥ 1 metabolic abnormality (e.g. hypercalciuria, hyper-oxaluria) but in most cases the cause of the abnormality itself is unknown.

Low urine volume is the most important predisposing factor to formation of calcium oxalate stones.

Calcium oxalate stones can exist at monohydrate (whewellite) and dehydrate (weddellite).

Calcium oxalate monohydrate stones are much harder to break – crystals are dumbbell shaped.

Calcium oxalate dihydrate crystals are pyramidal.

Hypercalciuria

Excretion of > 7mmol (men) or > 6mmol (women) of calcium per day

This increases SS of urine, and can be due to calcium:

- absorption (increased in intestine) seen in "absorptive hypercalciuria"
- excretion (leakage from kidney)
- resorption (increased de-mineralisation of bone)

The vitamin-D metabolite that stimulates intestinal calcium absorption is 1,25-dihydroxyvitamin D_3

"*Renal leak*" hypercalciuria is:

- renal wasting of calcium due to impairment of renal tubular reabsorption of calcium
- leads to secondary hyperparathyroidism (low bone density)
- treated with thiazide diuretics (augments calcium reabsorption in proximal tubule)

Hypercalcaemia

Almost all patients with hypercalcaemia who form stones have primary hyperparathyroidism.

Hyperoxaluria

Increased oxalate in the urine can be due to:
- leakage (altered membrane transport leading to increased renal loss)
- over-production (primary cause in liver)
- absorption (increased oxalate absorption in bowel)

The primary site of intestinal absorption of oxalate is in the large bowel.

Enteric hyperoxaluria managed by calcium supplements (bind excess oxalate within intestine which is soluble), potassium citrate (inhibitor of stone formation) and increase fluid intake.

Hyper-oxaluria is the most common urinary finding in patients with gastric bypass surgery.

Intestinal oxalate absorption is modulated by diet – low dietary calcium increases oxalate absorption due to reduced formation of soluble calcium-oxalate complex lost in stool.

O.formigenes is an oxalate-degrading bacterium found in intestinal lumen that uses oxalate as energy source, thereby reducing its absorption and thus urinary oxalate.

Aetiology of stone formation in cystic fibrosis patients is due to reduced / absent O.formigenes.

In inflammatory bowel disease the intestinal fat malabsorption increases calcium soap formation, limiting the amount free to complex with oxalate which in turn is free for absoprtion. [5]

Other

Hypo-citraturia, as citrate is stone-inhibitor (causes include renal tubular acidosis, hypokalaemia).

Hyper-uricosuria, high urinary uric acid levels

URIC ACID STONES

Approximately 50% of patients with uric acid stones have gout (20% of gout patients get stones).

The rest are idiopathic or due to myeloproliferative disorders and their cytotoxic treatment (cell necrosis releases large amounts of nucleic acids converted to uric acid).

STONES: BROAD PRINCIPLES

There are no known inhibitors of uric acid crystallisation.

Urine is SS with insoluble uric acid.

Uric acid exists in two forms in urine – uric acid (insoluble) and sodium urate (20x more soluble).

As the pH rises the proportion of uric acid as sodium urate increases, thus increasing the overall solubility (i.e. acidic low pH urine predisposes to uric acid stone formation).

Uric acid stones are the only ones that can be dissolved by medical agents (e.g. potassium citrate).

Potassium citrate is preferred as alkalinising agent (rather than sodium bicarbonate) as the sodium may inhibit calcium reabsorption, leading to hypercalciuria and thus calcium oxalate stone formation.

Diet is important in prevention – high protein / purine increases uric acid excretion and lowers pH.

Under light microscopy, uric acid crystals appear rectangular.

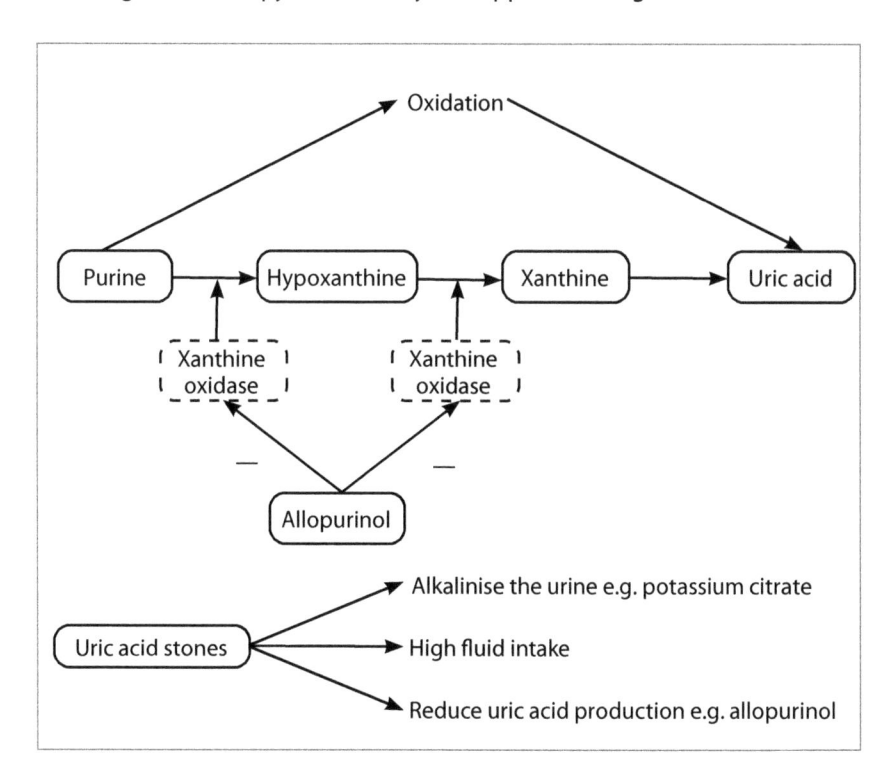

Figure 1 – Uric acid formation and summary of stone prevention strategies

STRUVITE STONES

Struvite stones are composed of magnesium, ammonium and phosphate (i.e. triple phosphate).

Urease-producing bacteria breakdown urea into ammonia, which alkalinises the urine increasing crystal precipitation of magnesium, ammonium and phosphate.

Struvite crystals look like "coffin-lids".

Acetohydroxamic acid is a competitive inhibitor of urease enzyme and can be given to prevent stone recurrence in patients with chronic urea-splitting infections.

Limited by side effects of DVT risk, hair loss and haemolytic anaemia [6]

IMAGING

Clinical situation will inform on most appropriate imaging modality, and if imaging (CT particularly) is negative then non-urological causes of abdominal pain should be suspected.

US URINARY TRACT

US is safe and inexpensive imaging tool – modality of choice in pregnancy and children.

US can detect stones in kidney, VUJ (with filled bladder) and upper tract dilatation.

Sensitivity for ureteric and kidney stones (45%)

Specificity for kidney (88%) and ureteric stones (94%)

NON-CONTRAST CT KUB (NCCT)

CT-KUB is standard for diagnosing acute flank pain (replaced IVU) and provides information regarding stone location, size, skin to stone distance, Hounsfield unit (HU) density.

Sensitivity is 94–100% and specificity is 92–100%.

No contrast is required (avoids risk of contrast reaction).

Quicker to perform than IVU, added benefit of being often able to diagnose cause of abdominal pain if diagnosis is not urolithiasis.

Indinavir stones and pure matrix stones (protein and cellular debris) are radio-lucent stones on CT.

Recommend scanning prone – VUJ stones that have passed into bladder will fall away from VUJ.

Standard CT KUB radiation dose is 4.7 mSv (IVU is 3 mSv).

[Natural incidence of fatal cancer is 1 in 5, but a 10mSv dose increases this by 1 in 2000, therefore a CT KUB by 1 in 4000].

An alternative option is ultra-low dose CT KUB (ULD CT KUB) which delivers 2–3 mSv, however at the expense of lower sensitivity.

CT Signs of Obstruction

The signs of obstruction on CT KUB include: [7]

- hydronephrosis and / or increased renal size (nephromegaly)
- unilateral perinephric / ureteric stranding
- ureteric wall oedema / ring around the stone (*Rim sign*)

Hounsfield Unit

HU is a quantitative scale for measuring radio-density.

Zero HU is the radio-density of distilled water at standard pressure and temperature. The HU of other common substances in the body are shown in (Table 4).

Table 4 – Hounsfield unit values for different substances in the body [7]

Substance	Hounsfield Unit (HU) on CT
Air	-1000
Lung	-500
Fat	-100 to -50
Water	0
Kidney	30
Muscle	10–40
Bone	700 (cancellous) – 3000 (cortical)

HU have ability to predict stone composition and thus help determine effective management plan for treating individual patient.

Uric acid stones have low density (200–450 HU) and can be treated with urine alkalinisation.

Calcium-bases stones have higher density (≥ 1000 HU) making them more resistant to ESWL and more likely to require surgical intervention.

CT attenuation values prior to ESWL helps predict treatment success.

- threshold of ≤ 815 HU has significantly better stone clearance rates [8]

The attenuation values of common stone composition types are shown in (Table 5).

Table 5 – HU for different compositions of stones [7]

Stone composition	Hounsfield Units
Uric acid	200–450
Struvite	600–900
Cystine	600–1100
Calcium phosphate	1200–1600

XR KUB

Kidney-ureter-bladder radiography (XR KUB) should not be performed in addition to NCCT.

Sensitivity is 45% and specificity is 80%.

XR KUB can be useful in determining radio-opaque vs. radio-lucent, and valid tool for follow up purposes for radio-opaque stones.

MR UROGRAM

MRU cannot be used to identify ureteric stones, however it can provide information regarding the level of obstruction, hydronephrosis and renal parenchymal morphology. [9]

Stones may be visualised as filling defects.

METABOLIC EVALUATION

There is no established consensus as to how stone-formers should be evaluated metabolically.

Stone analysis (performed by infra-red spectroscopy or x-ray diffraction) should be performed in all first-time stone-formers.

One method is to determine patient's risk of recurrence after stone passage, such that high-risk patients undergo thorough work-up, whilst low-risk patients have abbreviated work-up.

Low-risk metabolic work-up includes:
- *blood tests*, UEs, serum urate / calcium / phosphate
- *urinanalysis*, including pH (high in infection, low in uric acid) culture and sensitivity for bacteria, microscopy for crystals
- *stone analysis*

Factors that may deem a patient to be at higher risk of recurrent stone formation:
- children,
- white ethnicity with family history
- black ethnicity
- history of gout, recurrent UTIs, bowel malabsorption, osteoporosis
- uric acid, cystine or struvite stones

High-risk metabolic work-up includes (in addition to low-risk work-up): [7]
- 24-hour urine collection
- dietary diary

24-hour Urine Collection

Discard first voided urine, them collect all urine including following morning first voided one.

Store at cool temperature to prevent spontaneous crystallisation, analyse as soon as possible.

Two 24-hour urine collections are recommended as standard:
1. bottle with hydrochloric acid (tests 24-hour calcium, oxalate, phosphate, citrate)
2. standard bottle (tests 24-hour uric acid, electrolytes, pH, urine volume)

PAIN RELIEF

NSAIDs are 1st line analgesic for acute ureteric colic advised by EAU (opiates 2nd line). [10]

NSAIDs have better analgesic efficacy than opioids, and are less likely to require rescue (further) analgesia in the short term. [11]

Opioids are associated with a higher incidence of vomiting compared to NSAIDs.

NSAIDs induce afferent arteriole vasoconstriction mediate by prostaglandins, which reduce diuresis, oedema and smooth muscle stimulation.

The addition of anti-spasmodics to NSAIDs does not improve pain control.

RETROGRADE STENT VS. NEPHROSTOMY

An infected obstructed kidney is a urological emergency.

The patient should be resuscitated in a systematic Airway to Exposure manner, adhering to the principles of Sepsis-6 protocol.

Broad-spectrum antibiotics should be administered as per local guidelines.

NCCT imaging should be obtained urgently to confirm the diagnosis of obstructing stone.

There are two options for urgent decompression of obstructed kidney:
- placement of retrograde ureteric stent
- insertion of percutaneous nephrostomy tube

Studies suggest the two methods are equally effective in relieving the obstruction / infection.

A study randomising 42 patients presenting with obstructing ureteric calculi and infection to either percutaneous nephrostomy or retrograde ureteric stenting: [12]
- time to treatment was comparable between the two groups
- time to normal temperature was 2.3 days (nephrostomy) vs. 2.6 days (stent)

The decision may be based on logistical factors, surgeon preference and stone characteristics.

Table 6 – Percutaneous nephrostomy vs. retrograde ureteric stenting [7]

Factor	Stent vs. Nephrostomy
Nephrostomy bag	None required for stent
Failure rate	Lower in nephrostomy (impacted stone during stent)
Injury to adjacent organs	No risk with stent, nephrostomy may injury bowel / lung / spleen
Resource / availability	Stent does not require radiologist
Urine output monitoring	Nephrostomy allows monitoring of output from kidney
Ureteric access	Available after nephrostomy, not stent

STONE TREATMENTS OVERVIEW

STONE OBSERVATION

The younger the patient, the larger the stone and the more symptomatic the stone is, the more likely that treatment will be recommended.

Staghorn calculi are not suitable for watchful waiting (mortality ≤ 30% due to renal causes) unless co-morbidity poses higher risk during surgery.

Further consideration is occupation (e.g. airline pilot, bus / lorry driver), patients may have to be radiologically stone free before they are allowed to work again.

Civil Aviation Authority (CAA) do not allow pilots to fly until they are stone free.

Employees should be encouraged to inform their relevant authority e.g. DVLA, CAA.

Kidney Stones

The natural history of small asymptomatic kidney stones remains unclear – thus remains debatable whether they should be treated or followed-up.

Period of observation appears to be safe initial treatment option.

Evidence is conflicting and based mainly on single-centre observational studies:
- (Glowacki et al.) followed up 107 patients for 31 months – symptomatic event only 32%, of which half passed their stone conservatively [13]
- (Dropkin et al.) followed up 110 patients over 3 years, finding only 24% symptomatic and 19% requiring surgical intervention [14]

Follow up regime in a dedicated stone clinic may be tailored to patient.

Ureteric Stones

The cardinal factors to warrant intervention are infection, intractable pain or obstruction

EAU 2020:
- ≤ 95% of ureteric stones ≤ 4mm in size will pass within 40 days [10]
- spontaneous passage probability for stone 5–10 mm overall is 47%

A period of observation is therefore recommended by EAU Guidelines in patients with small (defined as < 6mm) stones in the absence of infection, obstruction or pain.

Stones that have not passed within 2 months are unlikely to do so.

CHEMOLYSIS

Oral chemolysis requires alkalinisation of the urine with potassium citrate or sodium bicarbonate.

The urinary pH should ideally be 7.0–7.2, however at a higher pH it may be more effective at the expense of increased risk of calcium phosphate stone formation.

Uric acid and cystine stones are potentially suitable for chemolysis.

EAU 2020 recommends using chemolysis for uric acid stones > 5mm (and combining with tamsulosin if stones are larger and obstructing). [10]

Patients should be taught how to self-monitor their urine pH and adjust medication dose accordingly.

MEDICAL EXPULSIVE THERAPY

MET in the form of alpha-blockers (tamsulosin, terazosin, doxazosin are equally effective) is currently under debate.

MET is contra-indicated in obstructed / infected kidney.

Patient should be counselled regarding side effects of postural hypotension and retrograde ejaculation, alpha-blocker use is "off-label" and evidence for efficacy controversial.

No evidence supporting use of corticosteroids as monotherapy or in addition to alpha blockers.

EAU 2020 however still propose MET effective for larger distal ureteric stones (> 5mm). [10]

SUSPEND Trial (2015) [15]

Lancet article often quoted regarding evidence against using MET.

Recruited > 1000 patients with CT confirmed ureteric stones to tamsulosin vs. placebo vs. nifedipine (1:1:1) with primary outcome being need for treatment within 4 weeks (all groups 20%)

Concluded MET should not be offered.

Criticisms include end point (did not prove that the stone had indeed passed) and that the majority of stones were < 5mm and thus would have passed anyway.

Furyk et al. (2016) [16]

Randomised > 400 patients with symptomatic distal ureteric stones < 1cm on CT, without fever or renal impairment, to MET vs. placebo.

Primary outcome measure being stone passage on CT at 28 days.

No overall difference found, however 22% increased chance of passage if distal and > 5mm (NNT 4.5).

EXTRA-CORPOREAL SHOCKWAVE LITHOTRIPSY (ESWL)

Three methods of extracorporeal shockwave generation are commercially available:

- *electro-hydraulic* (high-voltage between electrodes in water generates expanding bubble)
- *electro-magnetic* (electrical current through magnetic field generates shockwave)
- *piezoelectric* (ceramic elements expand rapidly when high voltage applied)

There are no stones that are resistant to LASER fragmentation.

Pneumatic systems have higher risk of proximal stone migration during treatment.

XR, US or a combination of both can be used to locate the stone for ESWL treatment.

Contra-indications to undergoing ESWL include:

- pregnancy (potential effects to foetus)
- bleeding diatheses
- uncontrolled UTIs
- skeletal malformations / obesity / aneurysm in vicinity
- anatomical obstruction distal to the stone

The most difficult stones to fragment with ESWL are calcium oxalate monohydrate.

Side-effects of ESWL include:

- visible haematuria, pain and infection (10–50%)
- failure of treatment or need for further sessions (10–50%)
- steinstrasse obstruction
- pancreatic or lung injury (rare)

EAU 2020 does not recommend routine stenting prior to ESWL as it does not improve stone-free rates (SFR) or lower the number of auxiliary treatments. [10]

Routine analgesia is beneficial as it limits pain-induced movements.

EAU 2020 does not recommend routine antibiotic prophylaxis be prescribed unless bacteriuria, known infection stones, indwelling catheter / nephrostomy). [10]

Patients with pacemaker and ICD can be treated with ESWL.

There is no strong evidence to suggest causal link between ESWL and diabetes or hypertension.

Struvite stones must be fragmented completely to minimise risk of urea-splitting bacteriuria.

Efficacy of ESWL depends on:

1. Stone size: more effective for stones < 1cm diameter
2. Stone Location: less effective in lower pole stones and / or in calyceal diverticulum
3. Stone Composition: less effective in cystine or calcium oxalate monohydrate stones
4. Best practice: US gel optimises acoustic coupling lowering shock-wave frequency from 120 / min to 60 / min, reduces tissue damage and improves SFR
5. Anatomical: Increasing skin to stone distance reduces efficacy (> 10cm) seen in obesity narrow infundibulum (< 5mm) or steep infundibular-pelvic angle

URETEROSCOPY

Rigid URS scopes have tip diameters 7–10 Fr (working channel 3.4Fr) and can be used for the entire ureter, and should always be used alongside a safety wire.

Flexible URS scopes are smaller (distal tip < 9 Fr) and accommodate working channel 3.6Fr.

Holmium:YAG Laser is the most effective LASER to treat stones (solid-state pulsed laser) in URS.

Has a favourable safety profile due to controlled shallow penetration depth and water absorption characteristics (meaning reduction of energy reaching non-target tissue).

Laser energy is delivered down a fibre with diameter 200–360μm.

Smaller fibres (e.g. 200μm) allow greater flexibility and preferable to use for renal (lower pole) stones.

The zone of thermal injury is limited to 0.5–1mm from the laser tip.

No stone can withstand the heat generated from Holmium:YAG laser, however harder stones will take longer to fragment / dust.

URS and Laser most suited for stones < 2cm diameter (reducing efficacy as stone burden increases)

The following are a list of potential *indications* to undergo URS:

- failed ESWL or hard stones (cystine, calcium oxalate monohydrate)
- ESWL unlikely to be successful (lower pole)
- stone in calyces diverticulum or infundibulum (may require incising)
- obesity, horse-shoe kidney, patient preference, pregnancy

Laser Settings

There are 3 parameters important to consider when fragmenting stones.

- *frequency* (Hz), increasing (30–50Hz) aids dusting (low Hz yields larger fragments)
- *energy* (J), low J (0.3–0.6J) favours dusting, high J breaks up stone into larger fragments and increases risk of retropulsion
- *pulse width / duration* (μs), longer pulse modes (800μs) result in less retropulsion

The frequency multiplied by the energy gives the power of the laser.

Access Sheaths

Hydrophilic-coated ureteral access sheaths (inner diameter ≥ 9F) can be inserted via guidewire placing the sheath tip in the proximal ureter.

Allows easy multiple access to upper tract, improves intra-operative vision due to continuous irrigation and reduces operative time.

Access sheath insertion may increase the risk of ureteral injury (risk reduced in pre-stented systems).

Stenting After URS

Routine stenting prior to URS is not indicated – although when present (eg. emergency insertion) it facilitates URS, improves SFRs and reduces intra-operative complications.

Routine stenting after uncomplicated URS is not indicated and may be associated with higher post-operative morbidity (storage LUTS, UTI) without benefiting SFR (EAU 2020).

Consider overnight placement of ureteric catheter instead with similar benefits.

EAU 2020 recommend stent insertion in the following circumstances: [10]

- ureteric trauma during the procedure
- residual stone fragments > 2mm within ureter
- bleeding (clot colic)
- URS during pregnancy
- impacted stone cases / prolonged procedures / use of access sheath

PERCUTANEOUS NEPHROLITHOTOMY

PCNL remains standard procedure for large renal calculi.

Standard access tracts are 24–30Fr, however paediatric sheaths < 18Fr are available and becoming increasingly popular for adult use.

(mini-PCNL 14–20F, ultra-mini PCNL 11–13F, micro-PCNL 4.5–6.5F) [17]

Initially collecting system inflated via fluid from cystoscopically inserted ureteric catheter, followed by percutaneous needle into calyx, guide wire insertion and sequential tract dilatation.

CT imaging prior to surgery is essential to provide information regarding interposition of organs.

Lower pole access is generally favoured in emergency setting (e.g. nephrostomy insertion).

Upper pole access is favoured for PCNL as it provides straight line to PUJ and access to all calyces.

The following are a list of potential *indications* to undergo PCNL:
- obstruction distal to stone location (i.e. cannot use ESWL)
- patient preference for most likely single session of treatment
- anatomical considerations (e.g. obesity, horseshoe kidney, kyphoscoliosis)
- failed ESWL / URS
- stone size (> 3cm / staghorn, or renal pelvis > 2cm or lower pole stone > 1cm)

Contra-indications to undergoing PCNL include:
- uncorrected bleeding disorder, pregnancy, sepsis, poor kidney function, confirmed or potential malignant renal tumour (absolute)
- high risk for anaesthesia, anterior calyceal diverticulum (relative)

Common side-effects of PCNL include:
- pain, bleeding, infection / sepsis
- multiple puncture sites for access / failure to clear stones
- major bleeding requiring emergency embolization ($\leq$ 1%)
- injury to bowel / liver / lung
- major bleeding requiring nephrectomy (< 0.1%)

Supine vs. Prone PCNL

EAU 2020 does not express a preference between supine or prone positions as they are equally safe, the SFR are comparable and operative time similar. [10]

Table 7 – Comparison of supine vs. prone PCNL techniques

Advantage of Supine PCNL	Advantage of Prone PCNL
Patient positioning faster and less risk of injury	Wider area / more options for puncture
Reduced anaesthetic / cardiovascular complications	May reduce risk of visceral organ damage
Simultaneous retrograde access to collect system	Greater manipulation of nephroscope

Tubeless PCNL

Tubeless PCNL is performed without a nephrostomy tube, totally tubeless PCNL without nephrostomy or ureteric stent.

EAU 2020 recommend tubeless / totally tubeless PCNL for uncomplicated cases. [10]

Totally tubeless PCNL is associated with shorter in-patient hospital stays.

Routine nephrostomy tube placement will depend on various factors including:

- likelihood of 2nd look procedure / large residual stones
- single kidney
- significant intra-operative blood loss
- ureteral obstruction
- urine extravasation / bacteriuria / infection stones

Colonic Injury in PCNL

Signs of colonic injury may be mild due to retro-peritoneal location and containment.

A ureteric stent should be placed to decompress system, withdraw nephrostomy from intra-renal position to intra-colonic thus serving as colostomy tube (keep > 7 days).

Perform nephrostogram prior to tube removal to ensure no colon to kidney communication.

LOWER POLE CALCULI

BROAD PRINCIPLES

Stratified by stone size, lower pole stones (LPS) fare worse than other sites.

This is due to poor clearance of fragments from the dependent lower pole, as the disintegration efficacy of ESWL is not limited for LPS compared to other locations.

Obtuse angles are likely to be more favourable for ESWL clearance than acute angles.

Anatomical considerations may further limit the efficacy of ESWL for treating LPS: [18–19]

- steep infundibular-pelvic angle
- long calyx (> 10mm)
- narrow infundibulum (< 5mm)
- long skin-to-stone distance (> 10cm)

If there are negative predictors for ESWL, then PCNL or URS are reasonable alternatives.

MANAGEMENT

Not all LPS (or kidney stones) require treatment and many can be observed.

EAU 2020 *indications* for active stone removal for kidney stones include: [10]

- stone growth (> 5mm)
- symptomatic stones (pain, infection, haematuria)
- stones causing obstruction
- patient preference / occupation / comorbidity

Risk of symptomatic episode / intervention in patient with asymptomatic renal stone is 10% / year.

ESWL, PCNL or flexible URS (FURS) are available options for LPS requiring treatment.

LOWER POLE CALCULI

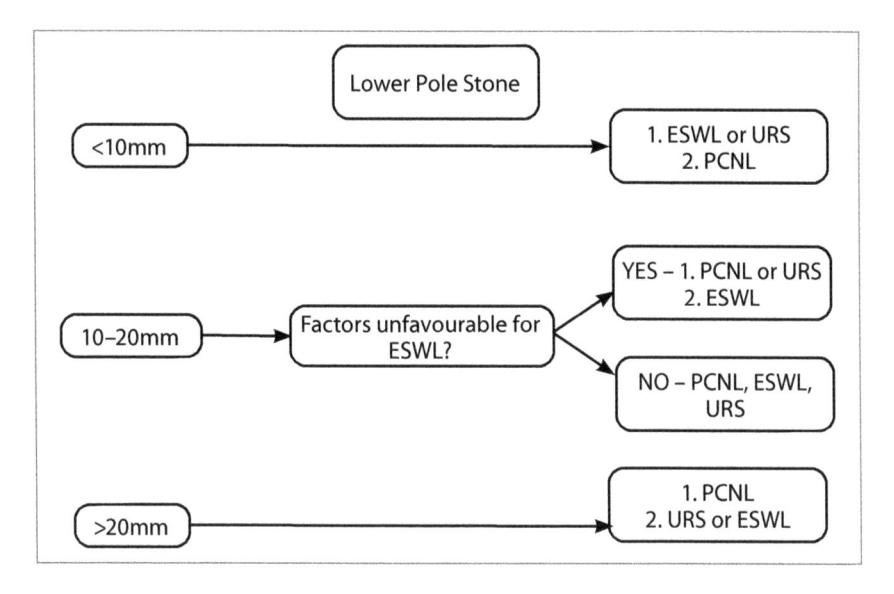

Figure 2 – EAU 2020 Lower pole stone treatment algorithm [10]

COMPARING TREATMENTS

Lower Pole I Study (2001) [20]

Prospective randomised multi-centre trial comparing PCNL (128) vs. ESWL (128) for LPS < 30mm

SFR at 3 months were 95% (PCNL) vs. 37% (ESWL)

Complication rates were 23% (PCNL) vs. 13% (ESWL)

Re-treatment rates were 11% (PCNL) vs. 31% (ESWL)

Main drawback of study was lack of comparison with FURS (addressed in Lower Pole Study II)

Lower Pole II Study (2005) [21]

78 patients with isolated ≤ 10mm LPS randomised to ESWL vs. URS

No statistically significant difference in SFR were found (although URS was 15% better SFR).

Greater operative time and complications were noted in URS group.

There is currently the PCNL, FURS and ESWL study (*PUrE*) undergoing in the UK to compare cost and clinical effectiveness of the different modalities of treatment. Results due.

URETERIC CALCULI

DIAGNOSTIC EVALUATION

Urinanalysis to evaluate for NVH should be performed.

Sensitivity for ureteric stones is 95% on first day of pain, and decreases over the following days, specificity is around 60%.

Always undertake a pregnancy test in women with abdominal pain of childbearing age.

The most important aspect of examination is temperature measurement – the presence of a fever may suggest an infected obstructed system which is a urological emergency.

MANAGEMENT

Patient should be resuscitated in a systematic Airway to Exposure manner, adhering to the Sepsis-6 principles where applicable.

Observation

Stone size is the main determinant of the success of conservative management.

Estimated that spontaneous stone passage rates ≤ 95% of ureteric stones ≤ 4mm in size

Observation is reasonable strategy for those who do not develop complications (infection, intractable pain, renal impairment) or have no social reasons to warrant intervention.

EAU Guidelines propose < 6mm ureteric stone should be regarded as "small".

Larger stones are unlikely to pass and should not routinely undergo a period of observation.

Irreversible loss renal function occurs within 2–4 weeks if completely obstructing ureteric stone.

Medical Expulsive Therapy

Please consult "Medical expulsive therapy" in "Stone Treatments Overview" station.

Retrograde stent vs. Nephrostomy

Please consult "Retrograde stent vs. nephrostomy" in "Stones: Broad Principles" section.

EAU 2020 advises that ureteric stents and percutaneous nephrostomies are equally effective: [10]

- key factor in choice is earliest intervention
- urine should be collected from drainage for culture

ESWL vs. URS

For practical purposes, ureter divided into thirds (proximal, mid-, distal) and patient is index (adult, non-pregnant, normal contralateral kidney, no comorbidities, no kidney stones).

For proximal ureteric stones:

- ESWL is superior for stones < 10mm
- URS is superior for stones > 10mm

For mid-ureteric stones both treatment modalities have equal efficacy.

For distal ureteric stones, URS is superior irrespective of stone size.

Overall the differences in SFR are not great when the two modalities are compared.

Many departments will not have 24-hour access to ESWL machine / technicians and therefore resource availability will impact management decisions.

PHYSIOLOGY OF UPPER TRACT OBSTRUCTION

Experiments carried out on dogs of the physiological response to complete ureteral occlusion yielded findings regarding the kidney's compensatory mechanisms.

FRCS (Urol) Part 1 MCQ may ask regarding the phases of response to complete ureteral occlusion

Phase I: (0–90 minutes)

Increased renal blood flow in response to rise in ureteral pressure, due to pre-glomerular vasodilatation.

Compensatory mechanism to increase capillary hydrostatic pressure / GFR

Phase II: (90 minutes – 5 hours)

Reduction in renal blood flow despite continued rise in ureteral pressure, due to post-glomerular vasoconstriction (further attempt by kidney to maintain GFR)

Phase III: (> 5 hours)

Fall in both renal blood flow and ureteral pressure due to pre-glomerular vasoconstriction (mediated by eicosanoids, renin, angiotensin II)

STAGHORN CALCULI

EPIDEMIOLOGY

Staghorn calculi are result of recurrent infection, thus more commonly encountered in women, renal tract anomalies, spinal cord injuries, neurogenic bladder or ileal diversion. [22]

PATHOLOGY

Staghorn calculi are composed of struvite (magnesium ammonium phosphate) or "triple phosphate".

Struvite accounts for approximately 70% of their composition and is usually mixed with calcium phosphate rendering them radiopaque on both XR and CT.

The following conditions must be met for struvite stones to develop:
- alkaline urine pH > 7.2
- ammonia in urine
- UTI with urease-producing organisms (proteus, klebsiella, enterobacter) which hydrolyses urea to ammonium and CO_2

The FRCS (Urol) viva may ask you to draw the equation for formation of staghorn calculi.

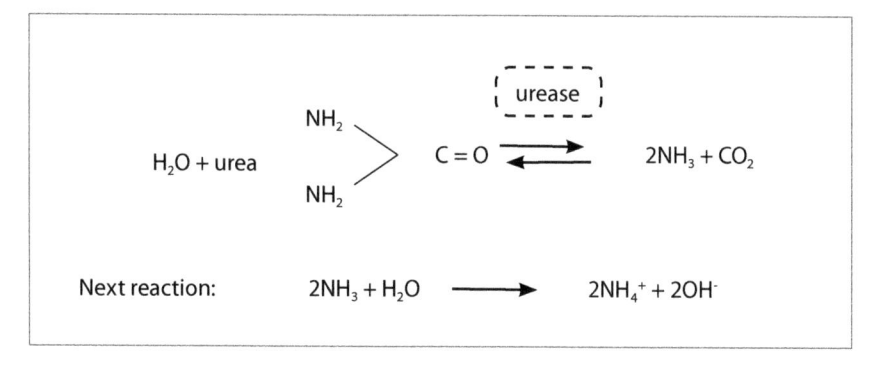

$$H_2O + urea \;\; \underset{NH_2}{\overset{NH_2}{>}} C=O \;\; \underset{\text{urease}}{\rightleftarrows} \;\; 2NH_3 + CO_2$$

Next reaction: $2NH_3 + H_2O \longrightarrow 2NH_4^+ + 2OH^-$

Figure 3 – Equation for formation of staghorn calculi

DIAGNOSTIC EVALUATION

Patients are deemed high risk and therefore should undergo thorough metabolic work-up.

DMSA is recommended prior to major surgical intervention, to obtain split kidney function which will ultimately determine management.

CTU is recommended to obtain a map of the calyces to plan optimal access to the kidney.

MANAGEMENT

Staghorn calculi should be treated surgically, provided the patient is anaesthetically fit and the affected kidney is deemed functioning on pre-operative DMSA.

Observation is no longer routinely recommended in patients fit for surgery. The FRCS (Urol) viva may ask you to quote evidence against the conservative management of staghorn calculi (see below).

The key principles in the management of staghorn calculi are:

1. Clear the stone (PCNL / URS) and infection (antibiotics)
2. High fluid intake
3. Consider acidifying the urine

Acetohydroxamic acid is a drug which competitively inhibits urease, and although it can help prevent stone recurrence its use is limited by side effects (risk of DVT, hair loss, haemolytic anaemia).

Blandy and Singh (1976) [23]

Article advocating a more aggressive approach to treating SC, in 3 parts:
- post-mortem study, 9/8996 post-mortems found a stag horn (and 5/9 died of related causes)
- retrospective study of 60 observed SC, where overall 17/60 died (28%), 20/60 had early nephrectomy and of the remaining 40, 16 developed pyonephrosis
- case series of 125 patients treated for SC (lower mortality of 7%)

Teichman et al. (1995) [24]

Retrospective analysis of 177 consecutive SC over > 7 years mean follow up

No patient with complete clearance died, 3% with residual fragments died and 67% of those who refused treatment died.

STONES IN SPECIFIC GROUPS

STONES IN PREGNANCY

EPIDEMIOLOGY

Pregnant patients do not appear to be at increased risk of stone formation compared to non-pregnant females of similar child-bearing age.

Urolithiasis affects 1 in 200 pregnancies.

Top reason for non-obstetric admissions during pregnancy is acute urolithiasis.

Occur most commonly in 2nd / 3rd trimester, associated with pre-term labour.

PATHOPHYSIOLOGY

The overall net effect of physiological changes do <u>not</u> increase risk of stone formation.

Factors promoting stone formation:
- physiological hydronephrosis and ureteric smooth muscle dilatation (progesterone)
- hypercalciuria (suppression of PTH)
- increased uric acid / calcium / oxalate excretion [25]

This however is counterbalanced by increased filtration of stone inhibitor citrate / GAG / magnesium. [7]

Physiological hydronephrosis is more common on the right (right 90% vs. left 10%) because:
- compression by dilated right ovarian vein
- uterine dextro-rotation
- protection of the left ureter by gas-filled sigmoid colon

Treatment not usually required for physiological hydronephrosis unless pain / sepsis in which case drainage should be considered (evaluate for obstructing stone as cause).

Physiological hydronephrosis will usually resolve within 6 weeks of delivery.

DIAGNOSTIC EVALUATION

Urinanalysis and MSU should be performed, FBC / UE / LFT / CRP measured.

Urgent review by obstetric team is mandatory.

Imaging

To avoid use of ionising radiation, EAU 2020 options in pregnancy include: [10]

- 1st line: trans- vaginal / abdominal US with full bladder
- 2nd line: MRI (if US equivocal, allows definition of obstruction level, view of other organs)
- 3rd line: low-dose NCCT with foetal shield, (avoid where possible)

US has poor sensitivity for ureteric stones (trans-vaginal may help with distal stones) and cannot differentiate between acute obstruction and physiological hydronephrosis of pregnancy.

MANAGEMENT

The patient should be resuscitated in a systematic Airway to Exposure manner adhering to the Sepsis-6 principles where applicable.

Multi-disciplinary approach recommended with shared input from obstetrics, urology, radiology

Pain Relief

Paracetamol and opioid analgesia are first line due to potential harmful effects of other drugs.

Avoid NSAIDs due to risk of closure of ductus arteriosus by blocking prostaglandin release.

Antibiotics

Antibiotic therapy should be based on available culture / sensitivity reports and local guidelines.

Prophylactic antibiotics should be considered as ≤ 50% of pregnant patients with stones have concomitant infection.

Penicillins and cephalosporins are considered safe in pregnancy.

Avoid trimethoprim (folate antagonist), gentamicin (auditory / vestibular damage) and nitrofurantoin (neonatal haemolysis).

Conservative Approach

Approximately 15–30% of pregnant patients with stones will need active intervention, ≤ 80% of ureteric stones will pass spontaneously due to physiologically dilated upper tracts.

Conservative management consists of rest, hydration, analgesia, anti-emetics and observation.

Patients with sepsis, intractable pain or renal impairment are not suitable.

Active Intervention

Percutaneous nephrostomy is beneficial in that it avoids GA.

Nephrostomy disadvantages include psychological implications of urine bag, dislodgement, recurrent blockages requiring frequent changes (every 4 weeks)

The alternative option is retrograde ureteric stent insertion.

Stent disadvantages include risk of GA, encrustation due to hypercalciuria requiring regular GA changes, irritative stent symptoms.

The surgical treatment of choice is FURS (modified dorsal lithotomy), however GA may induce pre-term labour and most would favour a delayed treatment approach.

EAU 2020 recommends non-urgent URS is best performed in the 2nd trimester. [10]

ESWL and PCNL are contra-indicated.

STONES IN CHILDREN

Children with urinary stones have a high risk of recurrence, and therefore a thorough diagnostic work-up should be undertaken.

Common non-metabolic aetiological causes include VUR, PUJO and neurogenic bladder.

> 1% of urinary stones occur in patients aged < 18 years.

Premature children are at much higher risk (increased oxalate excretion).

Hypercalciuria is the most common metabolic abnormality identified in children with calculi, and hyperoxaluria is commonly found in the context of CF. [26]

Imaging

Imaging in children may be challenging due to poor cooperation, always adopt the ALARA approach for radiation (As Low As Reasonably Achievable).

US with a full bladder is primary imaging technique in children (sensitivity < 60%).

If US inconclusive, consider low-dose NCCT as alternative.

Treatment Options

MET promotes stone passage but studies have not demonstrated efficacy / safety in children.

ESWL indications similar to those for adults, however children can pass fragments more easily.

- potential concern regarding ESWL safety on immature kidneys and surrounding organs
- need for anaesthetic has to be considered particularly in young children

ESWL remains the least invasive procedure for stone management in children and 1st line for single ureteric stones < 10mm or renal stones < 20mm.

PCNL indications similar to those for adults, as is the rationale for tubeless approach.

FURS indications similar to those for adults, benefit is lower radiation and in-patient stay compared to PCNL, however at cost of lower SFR.

STONES IN TRANSPLANT KIDNEYS

Transplant patients rely on their solitary kidney for renal function, and they are at greater risk of sepsis due to immunosuppression

Treatment must therefore promote immediate drainage.

Hyperfiltration, RTA and raised serum calcium (tertiary PTH) are stone formation risk factors.

Treatment Options

URS can be challenging due to anterior location of ureteral anastomosis.

ESWL is safe but stone-localisation is difficult and SFR are poor.

STONES IN CYSTINURIA PATIENTS

EPIDEMIOLOGY

Cystine stones account for 1% of adult stones and 6–8% of stones in children.

Peak incidence of stone formation is in 2nd to 3rd decade of life.

All cystine stone formers are deemed at high risk of recurrence.

Males and females are equally affected.

PATHOPHYSIOLOGY

Autosomal recessive pattern of inheritance leading to inborn error of metabolism. [27]

Patients can have homo- or hetero- zygous genotype, however the phenotype is the same.

Cystinuria is an inherited kidney and intestinal trans-epithelial transport defect for the amino acids (AA) cystine, ornithine, lysine and arginine (COLA).

Features reduced proximal tubular reabsorption of the COLA AA

There is excessive secretion of COLA in the urine, however only cystine is poorly soluble and so only cystine stones are formed.

Cystinuria patients often excrete > 1g of cystine a day (well above solubility of cystine).

Cystine solubility is low in acidic urine (hence the treatment strategy of alkalinising the urine) and will crystallise spontaneously in normal physiological urinary pH range.

Cystine crystals are hexagonal shaped.

Crystals are visible in only 25% or urine specimens, and therefore confirmation of diagnosis should be via 24-hour urine collection studies.

DIAGNOSTIC EVALUATION

Stone analysis is the optimal way to establish the diagnosis of cystinuria.

If stone sample is not available, use the 24-hour collection to detect crystals and measure urinary cystine levels, which can also help establish homo- vs. hetero- zygotes.

Brand's Test [7]

Also known as cyanide-nitroprusside test.

Cyanide converts cystine to cysteine, which binds to nitroprusside causing a purple hue within minutes if cystine level > 75 mg/L.

Over 24-hour collection test, homozygotes (>600 mg/day) and heterozygotes (200–400 mg/day)

MANAGEMENT

Surgical care is similar to that of patients with other types of stone, except cystine stones are more resistant to ESWL which may limit efficacy.

Medical care consists of a multi-modal strategy:
- *high fluid intake*, aiming for > 4L / day
- *urine alkalinisation*, aiming for pH > 7.5 (e.g. sodium bicarbonate, potassium citrate)
- *oral chelators*, bind to cystine as complex to increase solubility (e.g. Tiopronin / alpha-mercaptopropionylglycine (α-MPG))
- *captopril*, a 1st-line ACEi which also binds to cystine to form more soluble complex

α-MPG has similar efficacy to D-penicillamine (which binds to cysteine) in reducing urinary cystine but is far less toxic.

STONES IN HORSESHOE KIDNEYS

The prevalence of horseshoe kidneys is 1 in 400.

Due to abnormal medial fusion of meta-nephric blastema causing failure of ascent (by inferior mesenteric artery) and kidney rotation

Horseshoe kidneys are more caudal in position compared to normal kidneys.

The renal pelvis lies anterior to the calyces (all calyces are lateral to renal pelvis in normal kidney) and the calyces face posteriorly and caudally.

MANAGEMENT

ESWL

Visualisation may be challenging due to overlying bowel gas and / or bony landmarks.

ESWL can be successful however fragment drainage can be impaired by high insertion of ureter onto renal pelvis and relative urinary stasis.

URS

URS is a treatment option however likely need for flexible scope due to tortuous ureteric anatomy.

High SFR are achievable, however not matching those obtained in normal kidneys.

PCNL

Large stones > 2cm or in cases of failed ESWL / URS, then PCNL should be considered.

Tract difficulties include greater length, more medial location (higher risk of colonic injury) but lower chance of lung injury.

Usual point of access in horseshoe kidneys is the upper pole posterior calyx.

STONES IN CALCYCEAL DIVERTICULAE

A calyceal diverticulum is a non-secretory urothelial-lined compartment in (often very narrow) communication with the renal collection system.

Rationale for treatment vs. observation are the same.

For those requiring treatment, ESWL has low SFR due to poor drainage of fragments through the narrow communication point.

URS can be beneficial as it occasionally allows simultaneous incision of the diverticular neck.

PCNL is superior at obliterating the diverticulum and achieving greater SFR.

STONES IN RENAL TUBULAR ACIDOSIS

RTA is a defect of renal tubular H+ excretion – impairing ability to acidify urine (pH > 5.8).

The reduced ions will reduce bicarbonate reabsorption, promoting chloride reabsorption which leads to hyperchloraemic metabolic acidosis.

This serum parameter will promote resorption of bone apatite to raise serum calcium.

Hypercalciuria ensues, which further promotes stone formation in the alkaline environment.

Confirmation of diagnosis is via ammonium chloride loading test.

The most appropriate treatment is potassium alkali (potassium citrate) as compared to sodium alkali it reduces urinary calcium (sodium alkali may increase calcium stone formation).

Type 1 / Distal RTA

Distal tubule cannot maintain proton gradient between blood and tubular fluid.

70% of such patients have stones (calcium phosphate / brushite) (and often nephrocalcinosis).

Type 2 / Proximal RTA

Impaired bicarbonate reabsorption in proximal tubule, increasing urinary citrate (protects against stones) and thus not a relevant condition in stone formers

URINARY TRACT INFECTIONS: BROAD PRINCIPLES

TERMINOLOGY

Urinary tract infection (UTI), inflammatory response of urothelium to micro-organism invasion, usually associated with bacteriuria and pyuria.

Bacteriuria, presence of bacteria in the urine (bacteriuria without pyuria suggests colonisation)

Pyuria, presence of white blood cells (WBC) in urine

Sterile pyuria, presence of WBC in urine with bacteriuria (e.g. TB, CIS, interstitial cystitis (IC))

Cystitis, syndrome of dysuria, frequency, urgency with or without suprapubic pain

Acute pyelonephritis, syndrome comprising of flank pain, nausea / vomiting, fever > 38°C

Chronic pyelonephritis, radiological diagnosis describing scarred, shrunken kidney which may or may not have resulted from recurrent infections

Uncomplicated UTI, occurring in a patient with structurally and functionally normal urinary tract

Complicated UTI, in presence of underlying anatomical or functional abnormality also including:
- all men
- pregnant women
- indwelling catheters or stents, immuno-compromised, renal disease,
- hospital-acquired infections

Isolated UTI, occurs > 6 months after the previous UTI

Recurrent UTI, episode after successful resolution of an earlier UTI at a frequency of at least twice in last 6 months, or 3x in last 12 months, sub classified:
- <u>persistent</u>, recurrent UTI caused by same organism
- <u>re-infection</u>, episodes of UTI caused by different organisms (> 95% of recurrent UTIs)

Unresolved infection, one that has not responded to treatment (eg. Antimicrobial resistance)

Pathogenicity, the ability of an organism to cause disease

Virulence, degree of pathogenicity

Opportunistic infections, caused by non-pathogens (commensals) due to weakened host defence

Bacteriostatic, agent which stops bacteria reproducing whilst not necessarily killing them (bactericidal agents kill bacteria)

URINANALYSIS

GENERAL APPEARANCE

There are different possible colours of urine with listed causes:
- *cloudy:* phosphaturia (commonest cause), pyuria
- *red:* haematuria, myo-/haemo- globinuria, rifampicin, chronic lead / mercury poisoning
- *orange:* dehydration, sulfasalazine
- *yellow:* normal, riboflavin
- *green/blue:* biliverdin, methylene blue, amitriptyline
- *brown:* urobilinogen, porphyria, metronidazole, nitrofurantoin
- *brown-black:* laxatives, melanin

The most reliable urine specimen for culture is supra-pubic urine aspirate (avoids introduction of urethral bacteria).

The most accurate test for evaluation of kidney infection is direct ureteral catheterisation sample.

URINE DIPSTICK TEST

Blood

Orthotolidine (a peroxidase substrate) on dipstick comes into contact with haemoglobin (contains peroxidase activity) leading to oxidation reaction and cells lysis on strip. [28]

Same reaction occurs with myo- and haemoglobinuria.

The resulting colour change on strip is <u>blue</u>.

False positives – (oxidising agents) exercise, dehydration, menstrual blood

False negatives – (reducing agents) vitamin C

Leucocytes

Neutrophils (in infected urine) produce leucocyte esterase

Leucocyte esterase causes hydrolysis of substrate on strip to produce indoxyl, which oxidises diazonium salt chromogen on strip to produce colour change <u>violet</u>.

False-positives – specimen contamination e.g. vaginal discharge

False-negatives – old specimen (leucocyte lysis), dehydration, vitamin C, urobilinogen

Sensitivity is 70–95% (not all patients with bacteriuria have pyuria)

Nitrites

Most Gram-negative bacteria (i.e. most common uropathogens) convert nitrates (present in urine) to nitrites (not usually present in urine).

Nitrites react with aromatic amine on dipstick to produce colour change <u>pink</u>.

Griess reaction (detects presence of nitrite ion in solution) takes 4 hours.

False-positives – contamination

False-negatives – Gram-Positive bacteria (e.g. Pseudomonas), vitamin C, urine in bladder < 4 hours

Specificity 90–100% (i.e. patient likely to have UTI) however sensitivity is 35–85%

pH

Average urine pH 5.5–6.5

Alkaline pH > 7.5 in context of UTI suggests presence of stones.

Certain organisms (e.g. proteus, klebsiella, pseudomonas) produce urease:

- catalyses urea → CO_2 + ammonia (ammonia raises urinary pH)
- alkalinity causes precipitation of calcium magnesium ammonium phosphate (staghorn)

Proteins

80–150mg of protein is normally excreted in urine daily.

Dipstick contains tetrabromophenol which turns blue with albumin (> 20 mg/dL).

False-negatives – dilute urine, high pH, non-albumin proteinuria (e.g. Bence-Jones in myeloma)

Glucose

In normal conditions almost all glucose should be reabsorbed at proximal convoluted tubule (PCT) unless renal reabsorption threshold is exceeded (glucose > 180mg / dL).

Glycosuria may occur after sugar-rich meal or in diabetics.

Double oxidation of glucose results in colour change; this is specific to glucose and not other sugars.

Specific Gravity

Measure of density of the substances dissolved in urine, depends on mass of dissolved particles.

The test strip only measures cation concentration.

Will be raised in dehydration and diuretics, reduced in overhydration or diabetes insipidus.

MID-STREAM URINE CULTURE

The preparation of an MSU sample involves for the following patients:

- circumcised men – no preparation (void > 100mL and then collect urine sample)
- un-circumcised men – retract foreskin, wash glans with soap, provide sample as above
- women – retract labia, clean peri-urethral area with soap, provide sample as above

Ideally analyse culture within hours, alternatively refrigerate and analyse within 24 hours.

For microscopy, 5–10mL of sample is centrifuged for 5 minutes to collect sediment.

For culture, 0.1mL is delivered onto each half of split-agar plate and cultured overnight:

- one half has blood-agar for Gram-Positive organisms
- other half has eosin-methylene blue (EMB) for Gram-negative organisms

The number of colonies (CFUs) is then estimated.

Asymptomatic bacteriuria in women is defined as $\geq$ 10cfu / mL on MSU without any symptoms. [29]

GRAM STAINING

Staining method to distinguish bacterial species into 2 groups: positive and negative.

GS differentiates bacteria by chemical properties of their cell wall by detecting peptidoglycan.

The GS procedure is carried out as follows:
- bacterial smear is stained on slide with crystal violet for 1 minute
- Gram's iodine added for 1 minute and then poured off and slide is washed with acetone
- slide is then washed with water and safranin counterstain

The cell wall containing peptidoglycan will remain violet colour (Gram-positive). [28]

BACTERIAL VIRULENCE VS. HOST DEFENCE

The characteristics of uropathogens allowing them to colonise a host are *bacterial virulence factors*.

They can be divided into factors:

1. Directed Against External Agents

Anti-microbial resistance, which can be chromosomal inherited, arise from mutations or be independent from chromosomes via plasmids

2. Directed Against the Host

Toxin production, enzyme production (e.g. urease), anti-humoral substance production

Adherence mechanisms, where bacteria adhere to vaginal / urothelial epithelium and initiate UTI uropathogens express active proteins called *adhesins* on their cell surface

adhesins can be in the form of fimbrae/pili or may be afimbrial

E.coli has well-known pili facilitating adherence including:

- *type 1*, associated with cystitis (mannose sensitive) (produced by all strains of E.coli)
- *p-pili*, associated with > 90% cases of pyelonephritis (mannose resistant)
- *s-pili*, associated with ascending UTI, sepsis, meningitis

Conversely a number of host defence mechanisms exist to fight against the development of UTI:

- antegrade flow of urine
- exfoliation of urothelial cells
- presence of intact GAG-layer
- commensal flora of vagina (lactobacilli lower pH by converting glycogen to lactic acid)
- Tamm-Horsfall protein (made by loop of Henle) binds type-1 E.coli pili prevent adherence

ANTIBIOTICS

Antibiotic stewardship aims to optimise outcome of infection prevention and treatment, whilst curbing overuse of antibiotics. [30]

Method of action of common antibiotics are listed in (Table 1).

Antibiotic prophylaxis for surgery should be given ≤ 30 minutes prior to start of the procedure.

Table 1 – Mechanism of actions of common antibiotics used in urinary tract infections [28]

Antibiotic	Action	Mechanism
Quinolones (e.g. ciprofloxacin)	Bacteriostatic	Prevent DNA replication by inhibiting DNA gyrase
Macrolides (e.g. erythromycin)	Bacteriostatic	Inhibit protein synthesis
Tetracyclines (e.g. doxycycline)	Bacteriostatic	Inhibit protein synthesis
Trimethoprim	Bacteriostatic	Prevent DNA replication by inhibiting dihydrofolate reductase
Penicillins (e.g. co-amoxiclav)	Bactericidal	Interfere with bacterial wall synthesis
Cephalosporins (e.g. cefalexin)	Bactericidal	Interfere with bacterial wall synthesis
Aminoglycosides (e.g. gentamicin)	Bactericidal	Inhibit protein synthesis
Nitrofurantoin	Bactericidal	Damages bacterial DNA

RECURRENT URINARY TRACT INFECTIONS

DEFINITIONS

rUTI are defined as > 2 infections in 6 months, or ≥ 3 within 12 months.

These can be complicated or uncomplicated (and lower and upper tract), however repeated upper tract infection should prompt consideration of complicated aetiology.

Bacterial persistence leads to recurrence within days / weeks usually by same organism.

Re-infection usually occurs after prolonged interval and often caused by different organism.

In men with re-infection, likely to have BOO (urine is sterile in-between episodes) and should be investigated with uroflowmetry, PVR and flexible cystoscopy.

In women with re-infection, functional / anatomical abnormality is unlikely however vaginal mucosal receptivity for uropathogen is increased predisposing them to rUTI.

RISK FACTORS

Some women who suffer with rUTI may be inherently more susceptible due to their increased epithelial cell receptivity for uropathogens.

ABO blood group antigen secretory status refers to ability of individual to secrete blood group antigens, which is part of innate immunity against infectious disease.

The trait of increased susceptibility to UTI is associated with HLA-A3 phenotype, Lewis blood group status (Le a-b-) and (Le a+b-), P blood group secretors and ABO non-secretors.

Table 8 – Age-related risk factors for rUTI in women [28]

Young and Pre-menopausal	Post-menopausal and Elderly
Sexual intercourse (promote colonisation)	Urinary incontinence
Use of spermicide (promote colonisation)	Atrophic vaginitis (low oestrogen) (promote colonisation)
New sexual partner	Increased PVR volume
Mother with history of UTI	History of UTI before menopause
History of UTI in childhood	Cystocoele
Blood group antigen secretory status	Blood group antigen secretory status

DIAGNOSTIC EVALUATION

Patient *history* should enquire regarding the following:
- distinguish between isolated or recurrent UTI, and upper or lower tract
- sexual history and relevant association of UTIs
- past urological history / factors suggesting UTI may be complicated
- fluid intake, use of antibiotics, wiping patterns
- pregnancy status and use of oral contraceptive
- past medical history / drugs / immuno-compromise status

Patient *examination* (with chaperone present) should evaluate for:
- any underlying anatomical predisposing factors (eg. Palpable kidney or bladder)
- female genitalia evidence of cystocoele, tissue oestrogenisation, prolapse

Urinanalysis should be performed followed by MSU culture and sensitivities.

Imaging includes XR KUB (looking for stones) and US urinary tract with PVR measurement.

MANAGEMENT

In the acute UTI presentation, antimicrobial therapy is recommended because clinical success is more likely compared with placebo.

The choice of antibiotic is guided by local guidelines, allergies, sensitivities and pregnancy status.

Nitrofurantoin 100mg (PO) BD OR Trimethoprim 200mg (PO) BD are common 1st line choices.

PREVENTION

If investigations revealed no reversible factors, it is not possible to ensure rUTIs will not return.

Prevention strategies aim to reduce the frequency of infections:
- ensure high-fluid intake
- post-coital voiding, wiping front to back, limit perineal detergent hygiene use
- encourage cranberry juice intake
- topical oestrogen to vagina if atrophic
- prophylaxis with D-mannose
- lactobacilli intake to restore natural bacterial flora

Topical Oestrogen

For example, estriol cream daily for 2 / 52, then twice weekly for 2 / 12, discontinue for 4 weeks and reassess

D-Mannose

Prophylaxis with D-mannose 2g daily dose can be effective in preventing rUTI.

Functions by inhibiting bacterial adhesion by increasing clearance of bacteria in the urine. [31]

Cranberry Juice

Cranberries contain proanthocyanidins which can inhibit adherence of P-pili E.coli to uroepithelial cell receptors. [32]

Suggested that cranberry juice can reduce infections by ≤ 15%.

ANTIBIOTIC PROPHYLAXIS

Low-dose long-term prophylaxis works by eliminating introital reservoirs of pathogenic bacteria.

Prescribed in the form of one tablet every night, options:
- trimethoprim 100mg (PO)
- cefalexin 250mg (PO)
- nitrofurantoin 50mg (PO)

Breakthrough infections should be treated with a different antibiotic (based on sensitivities) and prophylaxis resumed after acute treatment.

Consider rotating antibiotic every 3–4 months are trialling scheme for ≤ 12 months.

Screening for asymptomatic bacteriuria and providing antibiotic prophylaxis is not recommended in diabetics, neurogenic LUTS patients (e.g. MS) or those with indwelling catheters.

SELF-TREATMENT

In patients with good compliance, self-treatment with a short antibiotic regimen is an option.

Patients encouraged to take MSU sample prior to antibiotics and proceed:
- 3-day course at full therapeutic dose
- single dose for post-coital prophylaxis (if rUTI closely related to sexual intercourse)

EPIDIDYMO-ORCHITIS

Acute inflammation of the epididymis, often involving the testis, usually due to bacterial infection

Epididymitis can be acute, chronic or recurrent.

Affects all male age groups

PATHOGENESIS

Infection ascends from the urethra or bladder.

In sexually active men aged < 35 years, common pathogens are N.gonorrheae and C.trachomatis, where a urethritis ascends to infect the epididymis.

In older men and children, the most common pathogen is E.coli.

In older men the most likely underlying cause is UTI as a result of BOO – recurrent episodes of epididymo-orchitis should prompt a full LUTS assessment.

m.TB is a rarer cause of epididymitis where the epididymis feels like a "beaded cord".

Men engaging in anal intercourse more likely to have enterococcal infections (e.g. gonorrhoea). [29]

Non-infective causes of epididymitis include:
- idiopathic
- traumatic
- due to amiodarone, which accumulates in high concentrations in the epididymis causing inflammation either uni- or bi- laterally and will resolve on interruption of the drug

DIAGNOSTIC EVALUATION

Patient *history* should enquire regarding:
- time and onset of scrotal pain / swelling
- previous episodes and treatment / past urological history
- sexual history and previous STIs

Patient *examination* (main differential diagnosis is testicular torsion) should evaluate for:

- spermatic cord thickening and tenderness, rather than testicular findings
- scrotal erythema or swelling
- urethral discharge
- Prehn's sign (positive if hemi-scrotal elevation relieves symptoms suggests epididymitis)

Testicular torsion features acute pain and swelling localised to the testis, whereas epididymitis is mainly preceded by infective symptoms with pain and swelling confined to epididymis

If clinical diagnostic doubt remains, surgical exploration is mandatory.

Urinanalysis and culture should be performed.

If there is no urethral discharge for collection, then first voided urine for PCR to detect chlamydia.

US scrotum indicated, may show increased Doppler flow around epididymis (and testis).

- US can be repeated if patient fails to improve to evaluate for scrotal abscess

MANAGEMENT

Patient should be resuscitated in systematic Airway to Exposure manner adhering to the principles of Sepsis-6 protocol.

Antibiotic prescription directed by local guidelines and discussion with microbiologist.

Any suspicion / confirmation of STI should prompt sexual health discussion with the patient and contact tracing as required.

Doxycycline covers chlamydial infection (azithromycin 1g stat if allergic as alternative) and ciprofloxacin covers gonococcal infection.

- if likely STI, ciprofloxacin (PO) 14 days + doxycycline (PO) 14 days + ceftriaxone (IM) stat
- if STI unlikely, consider ciprofloxacin (PO) 14 days

Persisting / worsening symptoms should prompt sonographic assessment for scrotal abscess, which may require urgent incision and drainage.

Chronic epididymalgia may require epididymectomy, best outcomes are seen in patients with post-vasectomy pain.

ORCHITIS

Orchitis is inflammation of the testis, however it often occurs in conjunction with epididymitis.

Causes include mumps virus, m.TB, syphilis, auto-immune (granulomatous orchitis).

Mumps Orchitis

Mumps orchitis occurs in 30% of infected post-pubertal males, starting 5–7 days after onset of parotitis and can result in testicular atrophy. [33]

10% of cases are bilateral and can cause infertility.

Management is supportive including scrotal support, ice packs, NSAIDs.

Mumps is a notifiable disease within the UK.

FOURNIER'S GANGRENE

Fournier's gangrene is a type-1 necrotising fasciitis of the external genitalia and perineum.

Most commonly occurs in men

Overall mortality 20% (higher in diabetics, alcoholics and immuno-compromised)

PATHOPHYSIOLOGY

Infection most commonly arises from the skin, urethra or anorectal regions.

Synergistic microbial action such that multiple aerobic / anaerobic organisms are present, most commonly E.coli, often facultative organisms (e.g. Klebsiella, enterococci, clostridia)

Risk factors include:
- recent instrumentation / catheterisation / penoscrotal surgery
- diabetes
- LTC in situ
- reduced mobility, elderly and infirm, immuno-compromised

Infection spread is through local fascia, producing tissue necrosis and pus by anaerobes.

DIAGNOSTIC EVALUATION

Patient *history* must enquire regarding:
- time of onset and relative distribution of perineal changes
- risk factors including long term catheter, recent urological surgery, diabetes, infirmity
- patient continence

Patient *examination* should evaluate for:
- focused urological: perineal swelling, oedema, erythema, tenderness, palpable crepitus
- signs of necrosis or gangrene
- fever and vital parameters

Cultures should be taken from relevant sources (urine, blood, groin pus).

Arterial blood gases and FBC, UE and CRP should be obtained.

Fournier's gangrene is a clinical diagnosis and therefore imaging is not routinely appropriate for confirmation.

Fournier Gangrene Severity Index

Mortality from Fournier's gangrene can be assessed via the Fournier Gangrene Severity Index (Laor scoring system). [34]

This is a scoring system assigning points based on various parameters, including:
- Temperature
- Heart rate
- Respiratory rate
- Serum sodium / potassium / creatinine / bicarbonate
- Leucocyte count
- Haematocrit

MANAGEMENT

The patient should be resuscitated in a systematic manner as per Airway to Exposure protocol, adhering to the principles of Sepsis-6.

Adopt multi-disciplinary approach to liaise with critical care, microbiology and anaesthetics.

Broad-spectrum antibiotics should be given immediately with early involvement of microbiologist.

    (often triple: co-amoxiclav, metronidazole and gentamicin)

Glycaemic control should be closely monitored and optimised.

Patient should be transferred to theatre without delay:
- debridement of all necrotic tissue until healthy margins reached
- urinary diversion in form of SPC should be considered
- faecal diversion in form of colostomy should be considered if colonic perforation
- open wound should be left (with scheduled re-look within 24 hours)
- testes usually spared as their blood supply is independent and distinct

Long term healing is good, however may require involvement of plastic surgery team.

EAU 2020 report no known evidence of benefit of negative pressure devices to promote wound healing in Fournier's. [29]

PROSTATITIS

EPIDEMIOLOGY

Causative pathogen is detected by routine methods in only 10% of cases.

In acute bacterial prostatitis E.coli is the most common pathogen, in chronic prostatitis the spectrum is wider, in HIV / immunosuppression organisms such as m.TB or candida.

Chronic bacterial prostatitis where symptoms persist > 3 months.

Chronic bacterial prostatitis is the commonest cause of recurrent UTI in men.

10% of men with acute prostatitis will experience urinary retention.

Highest risk age groups include 20–50 years and > 70 years.

RISK FACTORS

Risk factors are those predisposing to genitourinary tract and prostatic bacterial colonisation:
- UTI / epididymitis
- TUR surgery / indwelling catheters
- prostatic stones
- immuno-suppression

DIAGNOSTIC EVALUATION

Patient *history* should enquire regarding:
- fevers, chills, rigors, general malaise
- perineal symptoms including pain, discomfort
- irritative urinary symptoms
- previous prostatitis / chronicity of symptoms / known urological history

Patient *examination* should evaluate for:
- lower abdominal tenderness or palpable bladder
- DRE for tender prostate (or fluctuant to suggest prostatic abscess)

Haematospermia in men in endemic TB regions should be investigated for urinary TB (ejaculate analysis however is not recommended for microbial investigations).

Prostatic massage in the acute presentation is contraindicated.

Blood tests for FBC, UE, CRP

PSA measurement adds no diagnostic information in prostatitis, and a delay of > 3 months should be allowed to expect PSA to normalise.

Blood cultures if patient is febrile, consider urethral swabs for STI screen.

Most important investigation in the evaluation of a patient with acute prostatitis is MSU culture.

Imaging

US urinary tract to evaluate for urinary retention, PVR and hydronephrosis

TRUS may reveal intra-prostatic abscess and / or prostatic calcification – if this is too painful or not available, consider CT abdomen / pelvis to evaluate for abscess or collection.

MEARES AND STAMEY TEST

Meares and Stamey 4-glass test is standard method of assessing presence of bacteria in the lower urinary tract in men presenting with chronic prostatitis.

Not often used in daily practice because of time and difficulty performing it

The test is performed as follows (patient to have full bladder and no ejaculations > 3 days: [28]

- (VB1) 10mL of first-voided urine (positive culture indicates urethritis / prostatitis)
- (VB2) 100mL of voided urine from bladder (positive culture indicates cystitis)
- (EPS) following prostatic massage for 60 seconds the secretions are collected from urethra (positive culture indicates prostatitis)
- (VB3) 10mL of voided urine after massage (positive culture indicates prostatitis)

Where cultures are negative, increased numbers of leucocytes per high-powered field (>10) on microscopy favours a diagnosis of CPPS.

EAU 2020 recommends using classification by NIDDK in which bacterial prostatitis is distinguished from CPPS (Table 9).

Alpha-blockers may have therapeutic value in patients with category III (not as monotherapy).

Category IV requires no further investigations or treatment.

Table 9 – Classification of prostatitis and CPPS as per NIDDK [29]

Type	Name and Description
I	Acute bacterial prostatitis
II	Chronic bacterial prostatitis
III	Chronic abacterial prostatitis – CPPS
IIIA	Inflammatory CPPS (WBCs in EPS / post-prostatic massage urine / semen)
IIIB	Non-inflammatory CPPS (no white cells seen)
IV	Asymptomatic inflammatory prostatitis (histological prostatitis)

MANAGEMENT

Resuscitation in systematic Airway to Exposure manner, adhering to Sepsis-6 protocol principles

Antibiotic choice is guided by local protocols and discussion with microbiologists.

- consider broad-spectrum penicillin and quinolones
- consider extended course of step-down oral option
- intra-prostatic injection of antibiotics is not recommended by EAU 2020

In event of prostatic abscess, trans-urethral / percutaneous / trans-rectal drainage are options.

CHRONIC BACTERIAL PROSTATITIS

Defined as bacterial prostatitis where symptoms persist for > 3 months, caused by rUTI

Symptoms include chronic perineal pain, rUTI, ejaculatory problems and voiding LUTS.

Symptom Questionnaire

National Institute of Health (NIH) developed the Chronic Prostatitis Symptom Index, contains 4 questions pertaining to pain, 2 regarding urination and 3 about quality of life.

MANAGEMENT

Antibiotic courses should be extended for 4–6 weeks of quinolones.

Consider alpha-blocker to promote smooth muscle relaxation.

Fully investigate the functional lower urinary tract (uroflowmetry, PVR) and ensure this is medically / surgically optimised.

KIDNEY INFECTIONS

DEFINITIONS

Pyelonephritis is an inflammation of the kidney and renal pelvis.

Uncomplicated pyelonephritis, defined as limited to non-pregnant, pre-menopausal women with no known functional or anatomical urological abnormalities

Pyonephrosis, infected hydronephrosis as pus accumulates within the renal pelvis / calyces

Peri-nephric abscess, develops as a consequence of extension of infection outside the kidney parenchyma in acute pyelonephritis.

Emphysematous pyelonephritis, acute necrotising pyelonephritis by gas-forming organisms

Emphysematous pyelitis, describes presence of gas limited to renal excretory system.

ACUTE PYELONEPHRITIS

EPIDEMIOLOGY

1–2 per 1000 women are affected each year (0.5 per 1000 males).

More common in pregnant (1–4%) vs. non-pregnant women, and will occur in 25% of all pregnant women with untreated bacteriuria. [35]

Most cases of acute pyelonephritis start off as lower urinary tract infections.

Most commonly due to bacterial infection of E.coli (80%) due to P-pili virulence factors.

Risk factors include diabetes, pregnancy, sexual activity, recent urinary tract instrumentation, VUR, urinary tract obstruction and indwelling catheters.

PATHOGENESIS

80% acute pyelonephritis due to E.coli, other organisms include enterococci, klebsiella, proteus and pseudomonas.

Any process interfering with ureteric peristalsis (i.e. obstruction) may assist in retrograde bacterial ascent from bladder to kidney.

Initially there is patchy infiltration of neutrophils and bacteria in the parenchyma, later changes include formation of inflammatory bands extending from renal papilla to cortex.

DIAGNOSTIC EVALUATION

Patient *history* should enquire regarding:

- preceding lower urinary tract symptoms / cystitis / recent antibiotic use
- loin pain and / or visible haematuria (to suggest urolithiasis)
- fever / chills / rigors
- previous pyelonephritis episodes / past urological history / known stone former
- underlying conditions that may compromise patient immunity

Patient *examination* should assess for:

- abdominal examination for supra-pubic / renal angle tenderness
- presence of fever
- vital parameters

Patients with acute pyelonephritis tend to be symptomatic for < 5 days prior to presentation, whereas most peri-nephric abscess patients are symptomatic for > 5 days.

Urinanalysis to assess for infection and / or NVH

Urine culture and sensitivities should be performed.

Blood tests to include FBC, UE, CRP and blood cultures

IMAGING

US urinary tract should be performed to rule out stone disease or urinary obstruction (any hydronephrosis should be further evaluated with CT).

Persistent / swinging pyrexia can warrant repeat US to evaluate for renal abscess.

DMSA is the most reliable test for diagnosing pyelonephritis however rarely used 1st line in UK.

CT KUB can be requested as 1st line if high index of suspicion of underlying stone pathology.

FOLLOW-UP

Routine post-treatment urinanalysis or cultures is not required in asymptomatic patients except in pregnant women with asymptomatic bacteriuria (clearance must be achieved).

PYONEPHROSIS

Pyonephrosis is infected hydronephrosis where pus accumulates within renal pelvis and calyces – any cause of hydronephrosis can lead to pyonephrosis.

Associated with parenchymal damage and loss of renal function.

DIAGNOSTIC EVALUATION

Patient *history* should enquire regarding:
- preceding cystitis / pyelonephritis symptoms
- swinging pyrexia, night sweats and persisting loin pain
- known past urological history / urinary tract obstruction

Patient *examination* should assess for:
- flank tenderness (suggesting underlying abscess)
- fever and vital parameters

Urinanalysis, urine and blood cultures, blood tests are indicated as per acute pyelonephritis.

IMAGING

US urinary tract may reveal hydronephrosis, fluid-debris levels or air in collecting system.

CT may show peri-nephric fat stranding, renal pelvis thickening.

MANAGEMENT

A-E resuscitation and Sepsis-6 protocols as per acute pyelonephritis.

The key intervention is the urgent percutaneous drainage of pus from the kidney.

PERI-NEPHRIC ABSCESS

Peri-nephric abscess develops as a consequence of extension of infection outside the parenchyma of the kidney in acute pyelonephritis and develops within Gerota's fascia.

This abscess may therefore result from:
- rupture of cortical abscess
- failure to drain to pyonephrosis
- haematogenous spread of infection from distant site

Risk factors include diabetes, immuno-compromise and obstructing ureteric calculi.

Causative organisms include S.aureus (Gram-positive), E.coli + proteus (Gram-negative)

DIAGNOSTIC EVALUATION

Patient *history* should evaluate for:
- fever, unilateral flank pain and UTI symptoms
- history > 5 days in length is expected (compared to < 5 days seen in acute pyelonephritis)
- pyelonephritis which is not resolving despite ≥ 4 days of (IV) antibiotics should raise the suspicion of pus accumulation in or around the kidney.

Patient *examination* should evaluate for:
- flank mass with overlying skin erythema
- hip extension may trigger pain (psoas spasm)

IMAGING

US or CT-U can identify site, size and extension of retro-peritoneal abscess.

MANAGEMENT

A-E resuscitation and Sepsis-6 protocols as per acute pyelonephritis

The key intervention is the urgent percutaneous (or open) drainage of pus from the kidney.

Nephrectomy may be required for extensive involvement or non-functioning kidney.

EMPHYSEMATOUS PYELONEPHRITIS

Rare form of acute necrotising pyelonephritis caused by gas-forming organisms, with radiographic evidence of gas within or around the kidney [36]

Usually occurs in diabetics (> 90% of cases).

Other associated conditions may be urinary tract obstruction, stones, impaired immunity.

High levels of glucose in poorly controlled diabetes provides an ideal environment for fermentation by enterobacteria, producing CO_2.

There is an associated overwhelming inflammatory response, and due to diabetic microangiopathy the end products are not transported away. [28]

EPN is most commonly caused by E.coli and klebsiella.

Overall mortality is 40%.

DIAGNOSTIC EVALUATION

Severe acute pyelonephritis (high fever, flank pain, urinary symptoms, sepsis)

Patient may present acutely unwell, or rather fail to respond and deteriorate despite IV antibiotics treating their AP.

IMAGING

US will demonstrate strong focal echoes, indicating gas within the kidney.

CT can help classify EPN:

- *type 1*, destruction > 1 / 3 of the parenchyma with either absence of fluid collection or presence of gas radiating from medulla to cortex (mortality 60%)
- *type 2*, destruction < 1 / 3 of the parenchyma, confined intra-renal gas pattern, presence of renal / peri-renal gas within the collecting system, intra / extra renal collections may be present (mortality 20%)

DMSA scan is likely to show a poorly- or non- functioning affected kidney.

MANAGEMENT

A-E resuscitation and Sepsis-6 protocols as per acute pyelonephritis – early liaison with critical care and microbiology

Patients are usually very unwell at presentation and after resuscitation will require transfer to HDU /ITU for support.

Mainstay of management is supportive, antibiotics, fluids and percutaneous drainage.

If patient fails to improve, consider repeat CT in view of draining other pockets of infection.

Further deterioration may necessitate consideration of emergency nephrectomy.

XANTHOGRANULOMATOUS PYELONEPHRITIS

XGP is a severe renal infection resulting in diffuse parenchymal destruction and non-functioning kidney, usually associated with calculi. [37]

Proteus is the most common causative organism (E.coli also common)

Occurs more often in women

PATHOLOGY

Microscopically appears as diffuse infiltration of inflammatory cells (e.g. Lymphocytes, giant cells) and the characteristic finding of xanthoma cells (lipid-laden macrophages)

Macroscopically appears as enlarged kidney with yellow nodules of pus and areas of necrosis.

Radiologically difficult to discern from RCC and therefore clarity often only by histological analysis.

DIAGNOSTIC EVALUATION

Patient may present with flank pain, fever, visible haematuria and tender flank mass.

Complications include fistulae (nephrocolonic, nephrocutaneous), psoas abscess.

Blood tests to include FBC, UE, CRP, INR (likely to require percutaneous drain) and cultures

Urine culture (proteus more common than E.coli)

IMAGING

US will reveal enlarged kidney with echogenic material.

CT is investigation of choice, to identify cortical thinning, peri-nephric fat inflammation, hydronephrosis and nephrolithiasis ("bear paw abnormality"). [38]

DMSA likely to reveal poorly- or non- functioning kidney

CHRONIC PELVIC PAIN

CPPS is chronic or persistent pain perceived in structures related to the pelvis in men and women, where there is no proven local pathology / infection to account for symptom.

CPPS often associated with negative cognitive, behavioural, sexual and emotional consequences

Aetiology of CPPS is poorly understood and likely multi-factorial, including low-grade infection, chemical irritation, altered immunity and neuromuscular disturbances.

DIAGNOSTIC EVALUATION

Patient *history* should enquire regarding:
- duration of symptoms, impact on QOL, most bothersome symptoms
- previous medical or surgical treatments for condition (or pelvic conditions)
- urinary / bowel / sexual symptoms
- psychological well-being and history

Formal evaluation with Chronic Prostatitis Symptom Index questionnaire is encouraged.

Patient *examination* (with chaperone present) should evaluate:
- abdominal examination for anatomical abnormality (palpable kidney / bladder)
- DRE for prostate pain / tenderness
- external genitalia for scrotal pain / tenderness

Baseline urinanalysis and MSU culture and sensitivities should be performed.

Further investigations are guided by symptoms (e.g. uroflowmetry, urodynamics, cystoscopy, TRUS, semen analysis, STI screen).

Potassium chloride sensitivity test (Parson's test) consists of instilling potassium chloride into bladder via catheter, which may yield pain / cystitis symptoms (gauges permeability of GAG layer).

This test alone has a poor sensitivity and specificity. [39]

UPOINTS

UPOINT system is another tool to classify patients who have an established diagnosis of CPPS / PPS into a clinically relevant phenotype that can guide therapy.

UPOINT is not designed to diagnose these conditions.

(Urology, Psychology, Organ specific, Infection, Neurological, Tender muscle) [29]

PROSTATE PAIN SYNDROME

PPS is persistent or recurrent pain which is convincingly reproduced by prostate palpation.

The term chronic prostatitis is often used interchangeably however this is not appropriate.

PPS assessment should employ Meares and Stamey 4-glass test [discussed in "Prostatitis" station].

The diagnosis of PPS on the 4-glass test is established if:
- VB_1 (first-voided urine) and VB_2 (bladder urine) specimens are sterile
- EPS and VB_3 (post-massage urine) < 10,000 CFU bacteria and insignificant leucocytes

Presence of organisms / leucocytes in EPS or VB_3 specimens indicate possible chronic prostatitis

An alternative method is *Nickel's pre- and post- massage test* (PPMT), involving urine microscopy of pre- and post- massage samples (PPS possible if post-massage sample negative).

Classification

The classification of prostatitis is discussed in "Prostatitis" station.

TREATMENT

Cornerstone of management are antibiotics, NSAID and α-blockers.

Quinolones (e.g. ciprofloxacin) or tetracyclines (e.g. doxycycline) are particularly suitable for PPS as they show good penetration and bioavailability within prostate.

Start antibiotic + NSAID and continue for 4–6 weeks.

Do not use alpha-blockers as monotherapy or in treatment naive patients (try ≥ 3 months).

Alternative to NSAID (stop if no benefit in 6 weeks) are tricyclic antidepressants, diazepam or baclofen.

BLADDER PAIN SYNDROME

BPS is the presence of persistent or recurrent pain perceived in the urinary bladder region > 6 months, accompanied by ≥ 1 other urinary symptom.

There is no proven infection or other obvious pathology.

"Interstitial cystitis" and "painful bladder syndrome" are terms no longer recommended for use.

BPS is a diagnosis of exclusion.

Anti-proliferative factor is produced by bladder urothelium, potential mediator of BPS by increasing transmembrane permeability and decreasing heparin binding epidermal growth factor. [40]

CLASSIFICATION

Classification of BPS is based on cystoscopy and hydrodistension (+ / − bladder biopsy).

Glomerulations are pin-point red marks on bladder wall (petechial haemorrhages).

Hunner's ulcers are lesions described as circumscribed red area with small vessels radiating toward central scar with attached fibrin deposit and central fragility.

LASER fulguration of Hunner's ulcers can provide symptomatic relief.

Positive biopsy implies inflammatory and / or granulation tissue and / or detrusor mastocytosis.

MANAGEMENT

A holistic approach to the BPS patient is advised, working along a pain specialist, psychosocial counselling and support group.

Bladder instillations can be used to restore the GAG layer.

URETHRITIS

Urethral inflammation usually presents with LUTS, must be distinguished from other infections.

From therapeutic and clinical point of view, urethritis must be considered: [29]
- gonococcal urethritis (GU)
- non-gonococcal urethritis (NGU)

Other pathogens include C.trachomatis, mycoplasma genitalium, T.vaginalis.

Pathogens remain extracellularly on the epithelial layer or penetrate into the epithelium and cause pyogenic infection.

Chlamydia and gonorrhoea can spread further across urogenital tract to affect epididymis in men and endometrium and fallopian tubes in women.

Chlamydia is the most common STI in developed countries.

DIAGNOSTIC EVALUATION

Patient *history* should enquire regarding:
- dysuria, urinary symptoms, pain in penile shaft or meatus
- urethral discharge
- sexual history and previous STIs

Patient *examination* should evaluate for:
- external genitalia assessment for tenderness, rash, lesions or discharge
- fever and vital parameters

Perform MSU culture and sensitivity to rule out urinary tract infection.

Urethral smear diagnosis of urethritis:
- ≥ 5 polymorphs-nuclear leucocytes / HPF
- ≥ 10 polymorph nuclear leucocytes / HPF in first voided urine specimen

Collect 20mL of first-voided urine to test for chlamydia and gonorrhoea (NAAT).

Consider HIV and venereal screen testing.

MANAGEMENT

Patient should be resuscitated systematically in Airway to Exposure manner adhering to the principles of Sepsis-6 protocol.

Multi-disciplinary approach with involvement of microbiology and genitourinary medicine advised.

GU is treated with ceftriaxone 1g (IM) stat dose.

NGU is treated with doxycycline 100mg (PO) BD for 7 days OR azithromycin 1g (PO) stat.

If GU treated with single-dose therapy but patient does not improve clinically or symptoms recur within days, consider additional treatment for C.trachomatis (most common cause).

FOLLOW-UP

The main health risk associated with chlamydia is transmission to female partner, who will be subjected to risk of PID (10% risk if infected and untreated).

Informing GU department for contact tracing is important.

URINARY TRACT INFECTIONS IN PREGNANCY

EPIDEMIOLOGY

5% pregnant women have asymptomatic bacteriuria (same as background population of young women) however 30% of these will progress to develop pyelonephritis.

EAU 2020 – pregnant women should have asymptomatic bacteriuria treated. [29]

Short (2–7) course of antibiotics is recommended rather than routine prophylaxis.

MANAGEMENT

Antibiotic choice must bear in mind pregnancy status, allergies and anti-microbial sensitivities.

The safe antibiotics during pregnancy are penicillins and cephalosporins.

Antibiotics to avoid during pregnancy include:
- 1st trimester: trimethoprim (folate deficiency)
- 2nd and 3rd trimester: aminoglycosides
- all trimesters: quinolones, tetracyclines

Once treatment is complete a repeat MSU must be obtained and negative to confirm eradication, in contrast to uncomplicated UTIs where this is not necessary.

Recurrent UTIs in pregnancy – give low dose (125–250mg) cephalexin daily as prophylaxis.

URINARY SCHISTOSOMIASIS

EPIDEMIOLOGY

Urinary schistosomiasis is also called bilharzia.

Most commonly found in Africa, Asia and South America (second only to malaria in tropical countries with regard to economic impact)

PATHOPHYSIOLOGY

Schistosomiasis is caused by the parasitic trematode / flatworm called *Schistosoma haematobium* (other organisms include S.mansoni and S.japonicum).

Infection is acquired by exposure to contaminated water.

The parasites (cercariae) penetrate the skin of host, shed their tails and migrate to the liver to mature.

Adult worms then travel to veins of vesical plexus and lay fertilised eggs, which can:

- penetrate bladder and enter urine
- remain trapped in tissues and become calcified eosinophilic granuloma (T-cell response)

The disease has two main stages:

- *active*, when adult worms are laying eggs (eggs are immunogenic and cause symptoms)
- *inactive*, adults have died and there is a reaction to remaining eggs

Eggs are then shed to be uptake in fresh water by the intermediate host snail.

The intermediate host snail is specific:

- bulinus for *S.haematobium*
- biomphalaria for *S.mansoni*

You may be asked in the FRCS (Urol) viva to draw the life cycle of schistosomiasis (Figure 4).

Ureteric involvement complicates ≤ 25% of cases of bladder schistosomiasis, is usually bilateral and most commonly affects the distal ureter.

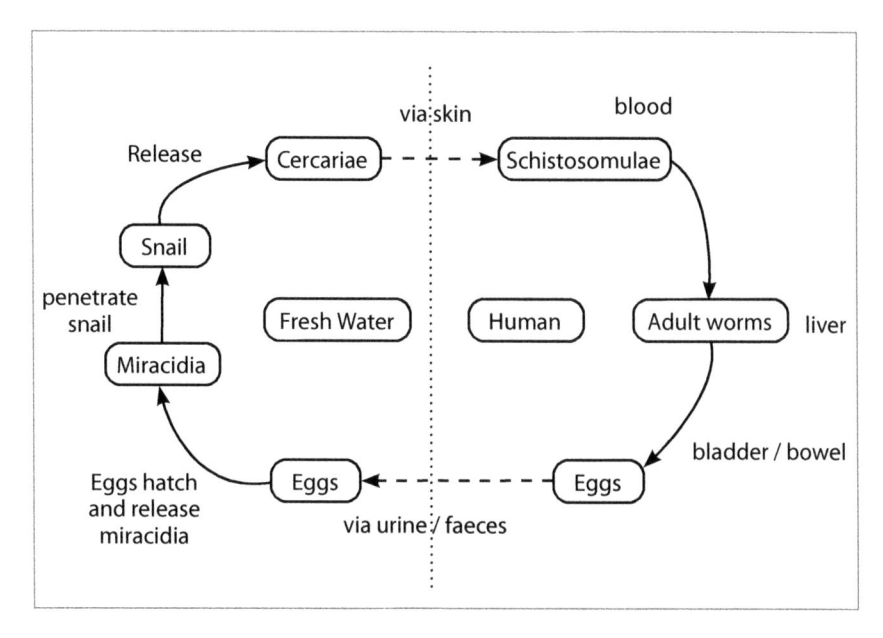

Figure 4 – Life cycle of schistosomiasis

DIAGNOSTIC EVALUATION

The first symptom may be dermatitis at the site of entry of parasite (swimmer's itch).

Followed by *Katayama fever*, a generalised immune reaction associated with onset of egg-laying to include fever, malaise, lymphadenopathy, hepatosplenomegaly (3–12 weeks)

Urinary schistosomiasis leads to visible haematuria (12 weeks) and terminal dysuria.

Blood tests

FBC reveals raised eosinophils.

UE will reveal raised creatinine in advanced disease.

Imaging

US may reveal hydronephrosis and / or thickened bladder wall.

CTU may show a calcified, contracted bladder.

Urine

Recommended <u>collection time noon – 3pm</u> to seek eggs (distinguished by terminal spine)

    (eggs may also be found in faecal sample)

More invasive tests include cystoscopy (sandy patches of eggs on trigone) or bladder / rectal biopsy to confirm presence of eggs.

TREATMENT

Praziquantel 40mg / kg as a single or divided dose (cure rate 85–100%) (if fails, repeat dose)

Steroids can be used to treat Katayama fever stage.

Patients should be followed up for clinical assessment, urinanalysis and consider cystoscopic surveillance (no agreed consensus for duration).

SEQUALAE

Chronic urinary effects include fibrosis, "eggshell" calcification of the bladder, reduced bladder compliance and subsequent hydronephrosis / high pressure system.

Increased risk of SCCa of the bladder

URINARY TUBERCULOSIS

EPIDEMIOLOGY

TB is predominantly seen in Asian populations.

Higher incidence in males compared to females [41]

The kidney is the most common site of extra-pulmonary TB.

In the genital tract, primary site of involvement is epididymis (males) and fallopian tubes (females).

PATHOGENESIS

TB of the genitourinary tract is caused by mycobacterium tuberculosis.

M.bovis, M.africanum and M.microti can also cause TB.

It is usually acquired in childhood by inhalation of infected droplets causing deposition of bacilli in the lungs (*Primary TB*).

In Primary TB, a granulomatous lesion forms in the mid-/upper zone of the lung; a central area of caseation necrosis surrounded by Langhans and epithelioid cells.

In immuno-competent individuals this process is self-limiting and sub-clinical.

Acute systemic dissemination of TB can however result in symptomatic *miliary TB*.

Post-primary TB is latent reactivation of infection which occurs at a time of host immuno-compromise, which will lead to clinical manifestations (25% of worldwide deaths in HIV patients is due to TB).

Life-time risk of TB reactivation is 10%.

The spread of infection from lungs to urinary system is haematogenous (to the kidney), from where by direct extension it can pass to ureters and bladder.

The pathognomic lesion of TB is the caveating granuloma.

This comprises Langhans giant cells surrounded by lymphocytes and fibroblasts, and the healing of these lesions causes fibrosis and calcification.

DIAGNOSTIC EVALUATION

Patient *history* should specifically enquire regarding:
- risk factors for TB – ethnic background, foreign travel, crowded accommodation
- symptoms of lethargy, weight loss, night sweats, fevers, haemoptysis
- UTI not responding to treatment
- other co-morbidities such as HIV, steroid use and diabetes mellitus

Patient *examination* should include:
- chest and abdominal examination
- any palpable lymphadenopathy
- genital examination

Urine dipstick will reveal sterile pyuria, no nitrites.

CXR may show granulomas, sputum culture should be sent.

Urine cytology to exclude other causes of sterile pyuria (e.g. CIS of the bladder)

Tuberculin Skin Test

Involves an intra-dermal injection of protein derivative of m.TB

A positive result suggests exposure to TB (not necessarily active infection) however a negative result excludes the diagnosis of TB.

URINE CULTURE

m.TB is not suitable for standard Gram-stain testing due to high lipid content of the cell wall.

m.TB is present intermittently in the urine and therefore sending multiple samples of early morning urine (has been stagnant in bladder) for analysis, minimises chance of false-negative yield.

The smear of the urine is tested using *Ziehl-Neelsen* stain looking for acid-fast bacilli (AFB) which will stain pink (non-AFB stain purple).

The specimen is also cultured using the Lowenstein-Jensen culture medium; however it is slow growing and may take 6–8 weeks to provide a result.

IMAGING

CTU is the radiological investigation of choice, as it allows visualisation of anatomy, strictures, calcification and parenchymal destruction.

CXR should also be requested looking for granulomatous lesions.

CYSTOSCOPY

Patients may have haematuria or voiding LUTS which warrant a cystoscopy.

TB of bladder may appear as areas of bullous oedema, ulceration and haemorrhage, and these can be biopsied and cauterised.

EFFECTS ON GENITO-URINARY TRACT

The first spread from the lungs is via the bloodstream to the kidneys, where it then may spread by direct extension to the rest of the urinary tract.

Kidney

Granuloma formation in renal cortex and caseous necrosis of renal papillae, leading to release of bacilli into urine.

Healing fibrosis and calcification leads to shrunken irregular kidney or "autonephrectomy".

Ureters

Ureteric strictures in TB are common.

Vesico-ureteric reflux is also common due to the distortion of the ureteric orifices.

Bladder

Spread to bladder is usually via kidney, however it can occur iatrogenically via BCG treatment.

Bladder wall becomes oedematous, red, inflamed (yellow lesions with red halo) and the characteristic fibrosis healing leads to small contracted, poorly compliant bladder.

Prostate / Seminal Vesicles

Haematogenous spread creates hard irregular calcifications.

Epididymis

Spread can be haematogenous or from kidney, lead to "beaded cord" which is usually unilateral.

Abscess and infertility are complications.

MANAGEMENT

The patient is best managed in a multi-disciplinary team setting with contribution from urologist, microbiologist, respiratory physician and local TB specialist.

Mainstay of management is multi-drug anti-TB regimens.

Typical combination is RIPE (rifampicin, isoniazid, pyrazinamide, ethambutol) for 2 months, and further 4 months of rifampicin and isoniazid.

(isoniazid causes peripheral neuropathy, rifampicin causes orange discolouration of urine)

Steroids not routinely indicated unless for ureteric stricture not responding to anti-TB medication

Multi-drug-resistant TB strains are becoming increasingly prevalent.

CALCULI AND URINARY TRACT INFECTIONS MCQS

1. Which of the following does not increase your risk of stone formation in urinary tract?
   A) Roux-en-Y gastric bypass
   B) high calcium intake
   C) testosterone supplementation
   D) horseshoe kidney
   E) corticosteroids

2. Which of the following is the best description of the shape appearance of uric acid stones under light microscopy?
   A) pyramidal
   B) coffin lids
   C) hexagonal
   D) rectangular
   E) dumbbell

3. Which of the following is the correct range of attenuation values (HU) for uric acid stones?
   A) 200–400
   B) 400–600
   C) 600–800
   D) 800–1000
   E) 1000–1400

4. Which of the following statements regarding the SUSPEND trial is false?
   A) Albeit not achieving statistical significance, the nifedipine group had marginally fewer patients requiring treatment within 4 weeks
   B) Adherence to medication was not assessed
   C) Patients with GFR < 30mL / minute were excluded
   D) Primary outcome was need for stone clearance treatment within 4 weeks of entry
   E) Patients were randomised to tamsulosin vs. nifedipine vs. placebo (1:1:1)

5. Regarding complete ureteral occlusion, which of the following statements is true?
   A) After 60 minutes there is decreased renal blood flow
   B) After 60 minutes there is no change in renal blood flow
   C) After 90 minutes there is post-glomerular vasoconstriction
   D) After 90 minutes there is post-glomerular vasodilatation
   E) None of the above

6. Which one of the following is not an amino acid whose transport defect is associated with homozygous cystinuria?
   A) lysine
   B) cysteine
   C) arginine
   D) ornithine
   E) all of the above

7. A patient undergoing investigations for prostatitis, has completed a Meares and Stamey four glass test. VB1 and VB2 have cultured negative, however VB3 culture reveals white cells. Which type of prostatitis as per NIDDK classification does this patient have?
   A) I
   B) II
   C) IIIA
   D) IIIB
   E) IV

8. Which of these antibiotics works by inhibiting DNA gyrase?
   A) ciprofloxacin
   B) doxycycline
   C) nitrofurantoin
   D) cefalexin
   E) tazobactam

9. Which of the following statements regarding the diagnosis of urethritis is correct?
   A) requires ≥ 20 polymorph nuclear leucocytes / HPF from urethral smear
   B) requires ≥ 50 polymorph nuclear leucocytes / HPF from urethral smear
   C) requires ≥ 100 polymorph nuclear leucocytes / HPF from urethral smear
   D) requires ≥ 5 polymorph nuclear leucocytes / HPF from first voided urine
   E) requires ≥ 10 polymorph nuclear leucocytes / HPF from first voided urine

10. Which of the following statements regarding bilharzia is incorrect?
    A) skin penetration occurs by cercariae
    B) areas endemic with s.japonicum have higher rates of seizures than baseline
    C) belongs to group of helminth infections
    D) ureteric involvement is normally to the distal ureter
    E) the name of the intermediate host snail for S.mansoni is bulinus

11. Which of the statements regarding urinary TB is incorrect?
    A) Gram positive organisms stain violet
    B) Lowenstein-Jensen culture takes ≥ 6 weeks
    C) spread to bladder features a yellow lesion with red halo
    D) pyrazinamide may cause peripheral neuropathy
    E) epididymal involvement is usually unilateral

12. What is the sheath size used in ultra-mini PCNL?
    A) 4.5–6F
    B) 7–10F
    C) 11–13F
    D) 14–16F
    E) 17–20F

13. Regarding the holmium:YAG LASER, the zone of thermal injury from LASER tip is limited to:
    A) 0–0.5mm
    B) 0–1.0mm
    C) 0–2.5mm
    D) 0–5.0mm
    E) 0–10mm

14. Which crystal shape best describes those of weddellite stones seen under light microscopy?
    A) pyramidal
    B) hexagonal
    C) rectangular
    D) dumbell
    E) coffin lid

15. Which of the following is an inhibitor of stone formation?
    A) pyrophosphate
    B) sodium phosphate
    C) magnesium phosphate
    D) potassium phosphate
    E) orthophosphate

16. Which of the following regarding renal leak hypercalciuria is false?
    A) urinary calcium loss occurs regardless of serum calcium levels
    B) urinary calcium loss is unaffected by dietary calcium
    C) serum PTH is raised
    D) it is associated with multicystic dysplastic kidney
    E) serum calcium is raised

17. Which of the following regarding staghorn calculi is false?
    A) staphylococcus heterogeneously produces urease
    B) they are more common in women
    C) mycoplasma is a urea-splitting organism
    D) acetohydraxamic acid is a direct antagonist of urease
    E) the crystal shape under light microscopy is coffin lid

18. Which of the following statements regarding urolithiasis and hydronephrosis in pregnancy is false?
    A) pregnant women have a higher excretion of magnesium vs. non-pregnant women
    B) pregnant women have a higher excretion of uric acid vs. non-pregnant women
    C) progesterone promotes ureteric smooth dilatation
    D) non-urgent URS is best performed in 2nd rather than 1st trimester
    E) nitrofurantoin avoided due to potential teratogenicity on foetal neurodevelopment

19. Which of the following statements regarding cystinuria is false?
    A) homozygous and heterozygous cystinuria have no difference in phenotype
    B) Brand's test relies on cyanide converting cystine to cysteine
    C) penicillamine can be used as an oral chelator of cystine
    D) crystals appear hexagonal under white light microscopy
    E) α-MPG is an oral chelator of cystine

20. What substance on a standard urine dipstick comes into contact with haemoglobin, which leads to an oxidation reaction and cell lysis?
    A) tetrabromophenol
    B) orthotolidine
    C) indoxyl
    D) diazonium chromogen
    E) sodium nitroprusside

21. Which chemical found in cranberry juice is thought to be responsible for its action in preventing rUTI in women?
    A) seminose
    B) proanthocyanidin
    C) GAG
    D) sodium hyaluronate
    E) u.ursi

22. Which of the following statements regarding mumps orchitis is true?
    A) seminiferous tubule necrosis occurs by pressure
    B) orchitis is more common in pre- rather than post-pubertal males
    C) the incubation period is 5–7 days
    D) mumps is a RNA adenovirus disease
    E) it causes oligospermia / azoospermia, but not asthenospermia

23. Which of the following best fits the description of category IV prostatitis?
    A) inflammatory CPPS
    B) chronic bacterial prostatitis
    C) chronic abacterial prostatitis
    D) asymptomatic inflammatory prostatitis
    E) non-inflammatory CPPS

24. Which cell type is characteristically found in XGP?
    A) acrophage
    B) polymorphonuclear cell
    C) lipid laden macrophage
    D) giant cell
    E) NK cell

25. Chlamydia trachomatis is:
    A) not a holoparasite
    B) facultative parasite
    C) Gram positive rod
    D) Gram positive coccus
    E) Gram negative coccus

REFERENCES

1. Reynard J, Brewster S, Biers S, (2009) Oxford Handbook of Urology 2nd Edition, Oxford University Press, Oxford.
2. Hyun JS. (2018) Clinical significance of prostatic calculi: a review. *The world journal of men's health*, 36(1), 15–21.
3. Ratkalkar VN, Kleinman JG. (2011). Mechanisms of stone formation. *Clinical reviews in bone and mineral metabolism*, 9(3–4), 187–197.
4. Evan AP, Lingeman JE, Coe FL et al., (2003). Randall's plaque of patients with nephrolithiasis begins in basement membranes of thin loops of Henle. *The Journal of clinical investigation*, 111(5), 607–616.
5. Hueppelshaeuser R, von Unruh GE, Habbig S et al., (2012). Enteric hyperoxaluria, recurrent urolithiasis, and systemic oxalosis in patients with Crohn's disease. *Pediatric nephrology*, 27(7), 1103–1109.
6. Williams JJ, Rodman JS, Peterson CM. (1984). A randomized double-blind study of acetohydroxamic acid in struvite nephrolithiasis. *New England Journal of Medicine*, 311(12), 760–764.
7. Johnston T, Rochester M, Wiseman O, (2018) Urinary Tract Stones. In: Viva Practice for the FRCS (Urol) and Postgraduate Urology Examinations, CRC Press, London.
8. Nakasato T, Morita J, Ogawa Y. (2015). Evaluation of Hounsfield Units as a predictive factor for the outcome of extracorporeal shock wave lithotripsy and stone composition. *Urolithiasis*, 43(1), 69–75.
9. Jung P, Brauers A, Nolte-Ernsting CA, (2000). Magnetic resonance urography enhanced by gadolinium and diuretics: a comparison with conventional urography in diagnosing the cause of ureteric obstruction. *BJU international*, 86(9), 960–965.
10. Turk C, Neisius A, Petrik C et al., (2020) EAU Guidelines for Urolithiasis. Available at: https://uroweb.org/guideline/urolithiasis/#1 [last accessed 31 May 2020].
11. Holdgate A, Pollock T. (2004). Systematic review of the relative efficacy of non-steroidal anti-inflammatory drugs and opioids in the treatment of acute renal colic. *BMJ*, 328(7453), 1401.
12. Pearle MS, Pierce HL, Miller GL et al., (1998). Optimal method of urgent decompression of the collecting system for obstruction and infection due to ureteral calculi. *The Journal of urology*, 160(4), 1260–1264.
13. Glowacki LS, Beecroft ML, Cook RJ et al., (1992). The natural history of asymptomatic urolithiasis. *The Journal of urology*, 147(2), 319–321.

14. Dropkin BM, Moses R, Sharma D et al., (2015). The natural history of nonobstructing asymptomatic renal stones managed with active surveillance. *The Journal of urology*, *193*(4), 1265–1269.
15. Pickard R, Starr K, MacLennan G et al., (2015). Medical expulsive therapy in adults with ureteric colic: a multicentre, randomised, placebo-controlled trial. *The Lancet*, *386*(9991), 341–349.
16. Furyk JS, Chu K, Banks C et al., (2016). Distal ureteric stones and tamsulosin: a double-blind, placebo-controlled, randomized, multicenter trial. *Annals of emergency medicine*, *67*(1), 86–95.
17. Wright A, Rukin N, Smith D et al., (2016) (2016). 'Mini, ultra, micro'– nomenclature and cost of these new minimally invasive percutaneous nephrolithotomy (PCNL) techniques. *Therapeutic advances in urology*, *8*(2), 142–146.
18. Manikandan R, Gall Z, Gunendran T et al., (2007). Do anatomic factors pose a significant risk in the formation of lower pole stones?. *Urology*, *69*(4), 620–624.
19. Sumino Y, Mimata H, Tasaki Y et al., (2002). Predictors of lower pole renal stone clearance after extracorporeal shock wave lithotripsy. *The Journal of urology*, *168*(4 Part 1), 1344–1347.
20. Albala DM, Assimos DG, Clayman RV et al., (2001). Lower pole I: a prospective randomized trial of extracorporeal shock wave lithotripsy and percutaneous nephrostolithotomy for lower pole nephrolithiasis—initial results. *The Journal of urology*, *166*(6), 2072–2080.
21. Pearle MS, Lingeman JE, Leveillee R et al., (2005). Prospective, randomized trial comparing shock wave lithotripsy and ureteroscopy for lower pole caliceal calculi 1 cm or less. *The Journal of urology*, *173*(6), 2005–2009
22. Diri A, Diri B. (2018). Management of staghorn renal stones. *Renal failure*, *40*(1), 357–362.
23. Blandy JP, Singh M. (1976). The case for a more aggressive approach to staghorn stones. *The Journal of urology*, *115*(5), 505–506.
24. Teichman JM, Long RD, Hulbert JC. (1995) Long-term renal fate and prognosis after staghorn calculus management. *The Journal of urology*, *153*(5), 1403–1407.
25. Semins MJ, Matlaga BR. (2014). Kidney stones during pregnancy. *Nature Reviews Urology*, *11*(3), 163.
26. Hoppe B, von Unruh GE, Blank G, (2005). Absorptive hyperoxaluria leads to an increased risk for urolithiasis or nephrocalcinosis in cystic fibrosis. *American journal of kidney diseases*, *46*(3), 440–445.
27. Claes DJ, Jackson, E. (2012) Cystinuria: mechanisms and management. *Pediatric nephrology*, *27*(11), 2031–2038.

28. Mishra V, Kalsi JS (2018) Urinary tract infections. In: Viva Practice for the FRCS (Urol) and Postgraduate Urology Examinations, CRC Press, London.
29. Bonkat G, Bartoletti RR, Bruyere F, et al. (2019) EAU Guidelines on Urological Infections. Available at: https://uroweb.org/wp-content/uploads/EAU-Guidelines-on-Urological-infections-2019.pdf [last accessed 31 May 2020].
30. Sanchez GV, Fleming-Dutra KE, Roberts RM et al., (2016). Core elements of outpatient antibiotic stewardship. *Morbidity and Mortality Weekly Report: Recommendations and Reports*, *65*(6), 1–12.
31. Kranjčec B, Papeš D, Altarac S. (2014). D-mannose powder for prophylaxis of recurrent urinary tract infections in women: a randomized clinical trial. *World journal of urology*, *32*(1), 79–84.
32. McMurdo ME, Bissett LY, Price RJ, (2005). Does ingestion of cranberry juice reduce symptomatic urinary tract infections in older people in hospital? A double-blind, placebo-controlled trial. *Age and Ageing*, *34*(3), 256–261.
33. Masarani M, Wazait H, Dinneen M. (2006). Mumps orchitis. *Journal of the Royal Society of Medicine*, *99*(11), 573–575.
34. Laor E, Palmer LS, Tolia BM, (1995). Outcome prediction in patients with Fournier's gangrene. *The Journal of urology*, *154*(1), 89–92.
35. Hill JB, Sheffield JS, McIntire DD, (2005). Acute pyelonephritis in pregnancy. *Obstetrics & Gynecology*, *105*(1), 18–23.
36. Huang JJ, Tseng CC. (2000). Emphysematous pyelonephritis: clinicoradiological classification, management, prognosis, and pathogenesis. *Archives of Internal Medicine*, *160*(6), 797–805.
37. Li L, Parwani AV. (2011). Xanthogranulomatous pyelonephritis. *Archives of pathology & laboratory medicine*, *135*(5), 671–674.
38. Lee JH, Kim SS, Kim DS. (2019). Xanthogranulomatous Pyelonephritis:"Bear's Paw Sign". *Journal of the Belgian Society of Radiology*, *103*(1).
39. Sant GR. (2002). Etiology, pathogenesis, and diagnosis of interstitial cystitis. *Reviews in urology*, *4*(S1), S9.
40. Kuo HC. (2014). Potential urine and serum biomarkers for patients with bladder pain syndrome/interstitial cystitis. *International journal of urology*, *21*, 34–41.
41. Figueiredo AA, Lucon AM, Junior RF et al., (2008). Epidemiology of urogenital tuberculosis worldwide. *International journal of urology*, *15*(9), 827–832.

STATION 6
UROLOGICAL IMAGING & PRINCIPLES OF UROLOGICAL TECHNOLOGY

MEASUREMENT OF GFR

UROFLOWMETRY

PRINCIPLES OF RADIOLOGY

NUCLEAR MEDICINE

OPTICS, SCOPES AND ACCESSORIES

STENTS AND CATHETERS

LITHOTRIPSY

THEATRE DESIGN, CLEANING AND EQUIPMENT

STATISTICS

MISCELLANEOUS

CONTENTS

MEASUREMENT OF GFR — 103
  MEASUREMENT OF GFR — 103
    CREATININE — 103

UROFLOWMETRY — 105
  ARTEFACTS ON TRACE — 105

PRINCIPLES OF RADIOLOGY — 106
  X-RAY PRODUCTION — 106
  RADIATION PROTECTION — 107
  CONTRAST AGENTS — 107
    IODINATED AGENTS — 107
    CONTRAINDICATIONS — 108
    GADOLINIUM — 109
  X-RAY KUB — 109
  DEXA SCAN — 109
  ULTRASONOGRAPHY — 110
    ULTRASOUND IN UROLOGY — 110
    DOPPLER ULTRASOUND — 111
  MAGNETIC RESONANCE IMAGING — 111
    CONTRA-INDICATIONS — 111
    DIFFUSION WEIGHTING — 112
    DYNAMIC CONTRAST ENHANCEMENT — 112
    APPARENT DIFFUSION COEFFICIENT — 113
  COMPUTED TOMOGRAPHY — 113
    CT UROGRAM — 114

NUCLEAR MEDICINE — 115
  MAG-3 RENOGRAM — 115
    RADIOISOTOPE — 115
    MAG3 TECHNIQUE — 115
    MAG3 INTERPRETATION — 116
    MAG 3 PHASES — 116
  DMSA SCAN — 119
    RADIOISOTOPE — 119

DMSA TECHNIQUE	120
PET SCAN	120
PET TECHNIQUE	120
UROLOGICAL APPLICATIONS	121
SINGLE-PHOTON EMISSION COMPUTED TOMOGRAPHY	121
RADIOISOTOPE MEASUREMENT OF GFR	121
STUDY TECHNIQUE [12]	122
NUCLEAR BONE SCAN	122
OPTICS, SCOPES AND ACCESSORIES	**124**
HOPKINS ROD-LENS SYSTEM	124
OPTIC FIBRES	124
SCOPES	124
ENDOSCOPIC INSTRUMENTS	126
STENTS AND CATHETERS	**128**
URETERIC STENTS	128
INDICATIONS FOR STENTING	128
METALLIC STENT	129
MULTI-LENGTH STENT	129
PROSTATIC / URETHRAL STENTS	129
URINARY CATHETERS	130
LITHOTRIPSY	**132**
ELECTROHYDRAULIC ESWL	132
ELECTROMAGNETIC ESWL	132
PIEZOELECTRIC ESWL	133
INTRA-CORPOREAL LITHOTRIPSY	133
SHOCK-WAVE PHASES	134
LASER LITHOTRIPSY	134
LASER SAFETY	136
THEATRE DESIGN, CLEANING AND EQUIPMENT	**137**
DEFINITIONS OF CLEANING	137
AUTOCLAVING	137
LEVELS OF DISINFECTION	138
THEATRE DESIGN	138

VENTILATION	138
THEATRE SAFETY	139
SUTURES	139
ENERGY IN SURGERY	140
MONOPOLAR DIATHERMY	141
BIPOLAR DIATHERMY	141
SAFETY	142
CUTTING VS. COAGULATION	143
HARMONIC SCALPEL	143
LIGASURE	143
STATISTICS	**144**
MISCELLANEOUS	**146**
BLOOD PRODUCTS	146
RENAL IMPAIRMENT	146
ACUTE KIDNEY INJURY	146
CHRONIC KIDNEY DISEASE	146
DIALYSIS	147
HAEMOSTATIC AGENTS	148
IRRIGATION FLUIDS	149
NOVEL PROCEDURES FOR BLADDER OUTFLOW OBSTRUCTION	149
REZUM® PROCEDURE	149
UROLIFT PROCEDURE	150
PROSTATE ARTERY EMBOLISATION	150
UROLOGICAL IMAGING AND PRINCIPLES OF UROLOGICAL TECHNOLOGY MCQS	**151**
REFERENCES	**156**

MEASUREMENT OF GFR

MEASUREMENT OF GFR

GFR is the volume of plasma filtered by the glomeruli in mL / minute.

Measured as clearance of any substance that is filtered but not actively secreted or reabsorbed by the tubules. Inulin is an ideal GFR marker but is difficult to assay in clinical practice.

Endogenous markers are used for daily practice, but exogenous markers are used if a more accurate measurement is required.

GFR is proportional to body surface area and is expressed as mL/min/1.73 m^2 (1.73m^2 being the average adult BSA).

Normal values are generally >90 mL/ min/1.73 m^2.

CREATININE

Creatinine is primarily filtered at the glomerulus, its production is relatively stable and hence it can be used as surrogate marker to calculate GFR.
[Image 1]

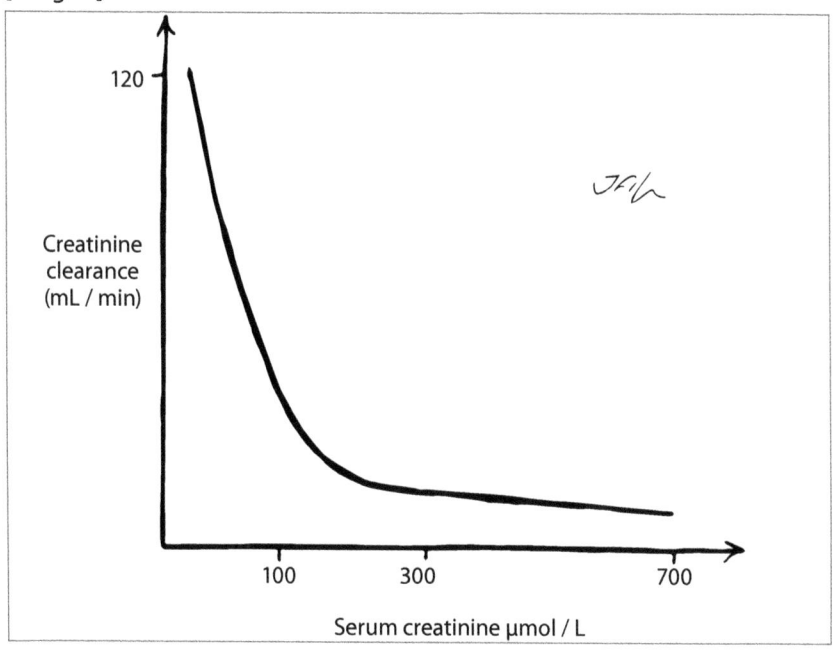

Image 1 – Relationship between creatinine clearance and serum creatinine

Graph suggests GFR calculation in relation to creatinine is less accurate as serum creatinine rises.

Creatinine tends to overestimate GFR when function is normal.

Creatinine is affected by muscle mass and is 10–20% is secreted by tubules.

Equations that can be used to estimate GFR include:
- Cockcroft-Gault formula – uses age, body mass and serum creatinine
- MDRD formula – uses age, gender, serum creatinine and Afro-Caribbean ethnicity (yes / no)

UROFLOWMETRY

Urinary flow rate estimation should be used as 1st line investigation of male patients with voiding dysfunction (less relevant investigation in women).

Uroflowmetry is a measurement of flow however provides limited inference regarding detrusor function.

Patients undergoing the test should have a normal desire to void and a voided volume > 200mL.

Currently, there are three established means of measuring urinary flow – spinning disc, weight transducer and capacitance. [1]

Each system has a funnel to collect urine, a flow measurement device and a means of data recording.

1. Rotating disc:

    Urine is directed onto a disc which spins at constant speed – the power required to maintain this constant speed is proportional to the flow of urine opposing the disc rotation. The volume can then be calculated by integration.

2. Weight transducer:

    Relies of gravimetric principle as the weight of urine collected indicates the volume and by differentiation the flow rate can be calculated.

3. Capacitance:

    As the patient voids and thus the height of the column of urine increases, the electrical capacitance of a bimetallic strip mounted in the chamber changes.

ARTEFACTS ON TRACE

Cough	short sharp spike of increased flow
Valsalva	wider increased flow spike
Wag / Cruise	patient mis-directing urine flow, causes flow spike with decreased flow either side
Occlusion	patients occludes urethra, flow goes to zero, urethra fills with urine and increased flow on patient release
Knocking	patient kicks device, high spike of flow which is very sharp and not physiological

PRINCIPLES OF RADIOLOGY

X-RAY PRODUCTION

X-rays are part of the spectrum of electromagnetic radiation, comprising of electric and magnetic waves travelling perpendicular to one another.

Their wavelength is shorter than that of visible light, in the order of 10^{-8} to 10^{-12} m.

Production of x-rays requires production of free electrons, which for purposes of clinical radiology occurs via heating a metal filament (the cathode) resulting in thermionic emission.

Electrons are accelerated in a vacuum toward a rotating metal anode where x-rays are produced.

X-ray beam is focused toward patient, who is placed between the x-ray source and a detector.

Tissues of different density cause attenuation of x-rays at different rates. Although x-ray attenuation is crucial to image formation, it is also a radiation dose to the patient.

Sievert – measure of health effect of low levels of ionising radiation on the body (the Sievert is often inconveniently large for various applications and so the mSv is used instead). It is intended to represent the stochastic health risk (see below). [2]

Gray – 1Gy is the radiation dose resulting in energy deposition of 1J / kg and tends to be used for higher doses of radiation that produce deterministic effects (see below) (e.g. dose of therapeutic radiotherapy).

Background radiation is 2–3mSv / year.

PRINCIPLES OF RADIOLOGY

Table 1 – Common imaging with ionising radiation and their equivalent radiation dose

Imaging Technique	Approximate Radiation Dose (mSv)
CXR	0.02
XR KUB	0.5
IVU	1–2
CT KUB	4–5
CT urogram	10
DMSA	0.001–0.4
MAG-3	2.6
PET	10

RADIATION PROTECTION

Radiation obeys the inverse-square law (i.e. if you double your distance from the source, the radiation will quarter) therefore keep as a great a distance away as possible.

Ionising radiation has two distinguishable types of effect on the body:

1. *Deterministic* effects, e.g. skin erythema and cataracts. There is a threshold dose below which no damage will occur. The severity of these side effects depends on the dose of radiation, dose rate, and number of exposures. [3]

2. *Stochastic* effects, e.g. carcinogenesis and mutagenesis. These have no threshold dose, as even a single exposure can result in damage. The frequency of stochastic effects increases with increasing dose, but their severity does not. They occur on random basis and is mutation effect.

CONTRAST AGENTS

Contrast agents are a heterogeneous group of pharmaceuticals used during radiological procedures to enhance tissue definition.

Three groups of intravenous contrast agents are available – iodinated agents, gadolinium and micro-bubble particles.

IODINATED AGENTS

Formed from organic acid salts of iodine

The relatively high molecular weight of iodine I^{127} makes it radiopaque.

When injected intravenously, iodinated agents are rapidly eliminated by renal excretion.

Iodinated agents are safe with generally low rates of adverse reaction (0.15%) e.g. nausea and vomiting, urticaria, skin rash.

Severe reactions are rare (<0.01%) and include bronchospasm, laryngeal oedema, and anaphylaxis (death rate estimated 1 in 100,000).

Contrast-induced nephropathy is a concern with iodinated agents.

The single most effective method to reduce risk of renal injury due to intravenous contrast, is ample intravenous hydration before and after the contrast scan is performed.

The American College of Radiology defines post-contrast AKI as ≥ 1.5x increase in creatinine from baseline within 48–72 hours. [4]

There is no absolute GFR below which contrast cannot be given – this decision will vary between different Trusts and radiologists.

A common approach is generally:

> GFR > 30 – proceed
>
> GFR 15–30 – equivocal
>
> GFR < 15 – do not proceed unless on dialysis

Patients with low GFR and on metformin must pause this the day before their scan, withhold 48 hours after the scan, re-start only provided GFR has not declined.

Poor metformin clearance may cause lactic acidosis.

CONTRAINDICATIONS

The Royal College of Radiologists state that increased risk of adverse reactions may be seen: [5]

- renal impairment
- previous adverse reaction
- asthma (avoid if patient is wheezy)
- diabetes and metformin therapy
- pregnancy

GADOLINIUM

The most widely used contrast agents for MR imaging are chelates of gadolinium.

Adverse reactions are low (0.04%), and serious anaphylactic reaction extremely rare.

Nephrogenic systemic fibrosis is a potentially fatal condition characterised by development of fibrotic tissue in skin and muscles due to accumulation of gadolinium in these tissues. [6]

There is no consistently successful treatment for nephrogenic systemic fibrosis.

X-RAY KUB

X-ray KUB is readily available, easily interpreted and will reveal the majority of stones (60–90%), however not uric acid, cystine (poorly) and indinavir.

Phleboliths appear rounded with a radiolucent centre.

DEXA SCAN

A DEXA scan is used to estimate BMD, which is used to diagnose osteoporosis / osteopaenia.

It works by emitting low dose x-ray beam with two distinct energy peaks (one absorbed by soft tissue and the other by bone), absorption subtraction can allow for BMD calculation.

Patient is supine, clothed (however no garments with metal), takes 5 minutes.

BMD score is compared with sex-matched to give WHO-defined T-score which is based on standard deviations from normal healthy adult.

    osteoporosis is < -2.5

    osteopaenia is between -1.5 and -2.5

    normal is > -1.0

Z-score is comparison of patient's BMD with age, sex, and ethnicity-matched reference data.

Z-scores are used in determining osteoporosis in young men, premenopausal women, children.

EAU (2020) recommends DEXA scan should be offered to men starting long term ADT to provide a baseline BMD. [7]

Osteoporosis in prostate cancer should be prevented with weight optimisation, regular exercise and ensuring vitamin D and calcium are within recommended levels.

ULTRASONOGRAPHY

An US wave is produced by the application of a voltage across a piezoelectric crystal which deforms, converting electrical energy into sound energy.

US propagated through body tissues at speeds which vary according to tissue composition.

When US hits interface between tissues it may be transmitted, refracted, absorbed or reflected.

Gel is used to reduce this attenuation occurring at skin interface.

Of the reflected sound a proportion will pass back to the transducer where the piezoelectric process is reversed; sound is converted to an electrical impulse which generates the image.

A grey-scale image is produced by returning echoes, the intensity determined by the strength of returning echo e.g. dense stone is white, soft tumour is grey, water is black.

The processes of absorption, refraction, and reflection are collectively termed attenuation.

Lower frequencies are used to look at deeper tissues (attenuation greater at higher frequencies).

ULTRASOUND IN UROLOGY

The following organs are visualised by US with their respective frequency:
- TRUS of prostate: 6–10MHz (prostate is close to probe)
- abdominal US: 3.5MHz
- testicular US: 7–12MHz

Therapeutic applications include ESWL and HIFU.

HIFU uses a frequency of 1–3.5MHz focused to reach high-intensity in thermal target area (cooling balloon protects rectal mucosa) to reach ≤ 90°C.

PRINCIPLES OF RADIOLOGY

Tissue damage occurs by coagulative necrosis – thermal injury and cavitation (microbubble formation and collapse). [8]

HIFU not currently recommended by NICE unless in context of clinical trial.

DOPPLER ULTRASOUND

Doppler principle is change in frequency (and thus sound) of a wave in relation to an observer who is moving relative to the source of the wave.

If the frequency of the transmitted beam is known and the frequency of the reflected sound is measured, the velocity can be calculated.

MAGNETIC RESONANCE IMAGING

Protons of hydrogen atoms usually spin in random fashion.

Upon entering an MRI scanner they align with the magnetic field in the longitudinal plane and produce a secondary spin (precession).

When a radio frequency pulse is applied the nuclei receive energy to move out of alignment and into the transverse plane.

When this pulse is removed the atoms release their energy in 2 ways:

- T1 Relaxation: energy released back into surroundings (realign back to longitudinal plane)
- T2 Decay: energy loss between adjacent nuclei

The release of energy is picked up as an electrical voltage by a receiver coil (MR signal).

Multi-parametric MRI combines anatomical sequences (T1 and T2) with functional sequences (DWI, DCE, ADC) to improve accuracy of prostate cancer diagnosis.

CONTRA-INDICATIONS

Strong magnetic fields around MRI scanner ensure that some special precautions are necessary.

Absolute contraindications include:

- metallic foreign bodies, e.g. metal in eyes from welding,
- cardiac pacemakers, cardiac devices, SNM devices
- ferrous containing aneurysm coils

T1 Image

T1 relaxation occurs more rapidly in fat (large molecules give energy back to environment quicker).

Fat appears very bright, while fluid remains dark, such that these scans are excellent for viewing anatomy due to the good tissue differentiation.

T2 Image

T2 decay occurs more slowly in water, resulting in higher signal.

Water has a very bright signal on these images, producing a scan which is more useful for demonstrating pathology (i.e. water appears white).

If during the FRCS (Urol) viva you are unsure as to the type of MR image you are being shown, look at bladder / CSF – if these are bright, image is T2.

Prostate appears dark / black in prostate cancer.

DIFFUSION WEIGHTING

DW-MRI imaging exploits the random motion of water molecules.

"Brownian motion" applies to water molecules in an unrestricted environment, the water molecules move in random motion.

This free movement of water is restricted in the body by boundaries formed by cell membranes.

Tissues typically demonstrating restricted diffusion include cancer, oedema, fibrosis and abscess.

Densely cellular prostate cancer displays restricted diffusion compared to normal adjacent peripheral zone tissue.

Prostate cancer appears brighter than normal peripheral zone tissue on DW-MRI.

DYNAMIC CONTRAST ENHANCEMENT

DCE measures blood flow in / out of prostate tissue.

In prostate cancer there is rapid wash in / out, and therefore will show early enhancement.

APPARENT DIFFUSION COEFFICIENT

The impedance of DWI water molecules can be quantified with an ADC value, which is calculated by software and displayed as a parametric map (prostate cancer appears darker).

COMPUTED TOMOGRAPHY

X-rays are produced when fast moving electrons are stopped suddenly by impact on metal target.

The kinetic energy of the elections is converted into x-rays (1%) and heat (99%).

An x-ray tube consists of two electrodes in a vacuum; the negative electrode (cathode, a fine tungsten filament) and the positive electrode (anode); a smooth flat metal target.

The filament is heated and emits electrons by the process of thermionic emission.

The electrons are attracted by the positive anode.

Each electron arrives at the target surface with a kinetic energy equivalent to the voltage (kV).

X-rays may be:
- transmitted: pass through unaffected
- absorbed: transfer to the matter some or all of their energy
- scattered: diverted in a new direction, with or without loss of energy

    Attenuation is the reduction in intensity of the primary XR beam as it passes through a medium.

    (attenuation = absorption + scatter)

In CT the x-ray beam is attenuated by absorption and scatter as it passes through the patient.

Detectors around the patient measure the x-ray transmission, these measurements are repeated many times from different directions as it rotates 360° around the patient.

Image is reconstructed, where transmitted x-rays are measured and assigned to each pixel according to the attenuation.

HU scale is used:
- water is assigned a value of 0
- the scale extends from -1000 HU for air
- to +3,000 HU for dense bone

CT UROGRAM

A CT urogram / urinary tract protocol sequence will vary between Trusts and radiologists, however a commonly used sequence includes:
- Initial non-contrast phase
- Arterial phase – 20 seconds (maximal enhancement of abdominal and renal vessels)
- Nephrographic phase – 70–90s (renal cortex)
- Urographic phase – 5–10 minutes (pelvicalyceal system, ureters, bladder)

Split-bolus technique is used to reduce the radiation dose.

Done via initial non-contrast phase, after this 50% of the IV contrast is given, wait 7–8 minutes and give other 50%. CT performed after 60s to combine both urographic and nephrographic phases.

NUCLEAR MEDICINE

Nuclear medicine scans rely on emission radiography – providing functional information by injecting a radioactive agent which is attached to a metabolite.

MAG-3 RENOGRAM

The MAG3 scan is a dynamic scan producing a video, from which images are then provided as a series of still photos.

MAG3 are most useful where there is concern regarding upper tract obstruction (e.g. PUJ).

The investigation also approximates differential function.

Glomeruli / tubules take ≥ 3 months to mature after birth – hence the recommendation that isotope renograms only be performed after this age.

The *diuresis renogram* is a variant of the standard renogram in which the urine flow rate is increased by administration of an intravenous diuretic (e.g. furosemide).

The diuretic response is proportional to the renal function and thus one should avoid interpreting or indeed performing MAG3 renograms in patients with eGFR < 15mL / min.

RADIOISOTOPE

The most commonly used radioisotope is metastable technetium-99 (^{99m}Tc).

The half-life of ^{99m}Tc is 6 hours. [9]

Approximately 90% of ^{99m}Tc MAG3 is cleared in the urine by tubular secretion and 10% by glomerular filtration (furosemide is given to ensure kidneys are maximally diuresing).

^{9m}Tc decays by emission of gamma rays only (not α or β).

Available from a generator which provides daily supply from decay of longer-lived parent ^{99}Mo.

MAG3 TECHNIQUE

The patient should be well-hydrated prior to the test.

Furosemide's maximal effect is seen at ~20 minutes – traditionally it was given 20 minutes after isotope (F+20) but this led to obstruction noted late in study and more chance of equivocal result.

Furosemide given 15 minutes prior to isotope injection (F-15) is now more commonly used.

Patient positioned either seated with back to gamma camera or supine with camera underneath.

After isotope is injected the gamma camera starts immediately:
- dynamic images taken every 2 seconds for one minute
- then every 20 seconds for 30–40 minutes
- patient asked to void at end of study and post-void image taken

MAG3 INTERPRETATION

On computer images of dynamic series, regions of interest are drawn around each kidney.

Activity / time curves are created showing how activity in each region of interest changes with time, and a background curve is used to subtract background contribution from each kidney curve.

The resulting curve is a renogram.

The relative function of each kidney is calculated from the uptake phase (1–3 minutes).

MAG 3 PHASES

The study begins with the vascular phase:
- occurs within first few seconds after isotope injection
- represents rapid flow of isotope to the kidney
- most of isotope is not extracted and remains in blood in kidney
- this phase should be removed from the renogram curve which should rise smoothly

1 minute onwards, renogram curve rises at rate proportional to kidney function (uptake phase).

3 minutes onwards, renogram curve may peak and begin to fall (elimination phase).

- this is a balance between elimination and uptake
- rising curve means uptake exceeds elimination (falling curve implies the reverse)

The diuresis renogram curves (O'Reilly's curves) for F+20 are exam favourites in the FRCS (Urol) viva and you may be expected to draw them (Figure 1).

- *Type I* – normal renal uptake and drainage
- *Type II* – obstructed pattern – no response to diuretic, curve rises or remains high
- *Type IIIa* – normal drainage but from hypotonic renal pelvis, falls rapidly after furosemide
- *Type IIIb* – equivocal, rises rapidly but neither falls nor rises after furosemide – this requires further evaluation, could be partial ureteric obstruction or impaired renal function
- *Type IV* (*Homsy's sign*) – furosemide causes transient response appearing decompensated at high flow suggesting likely obstruction, (F-20) is required to confirm

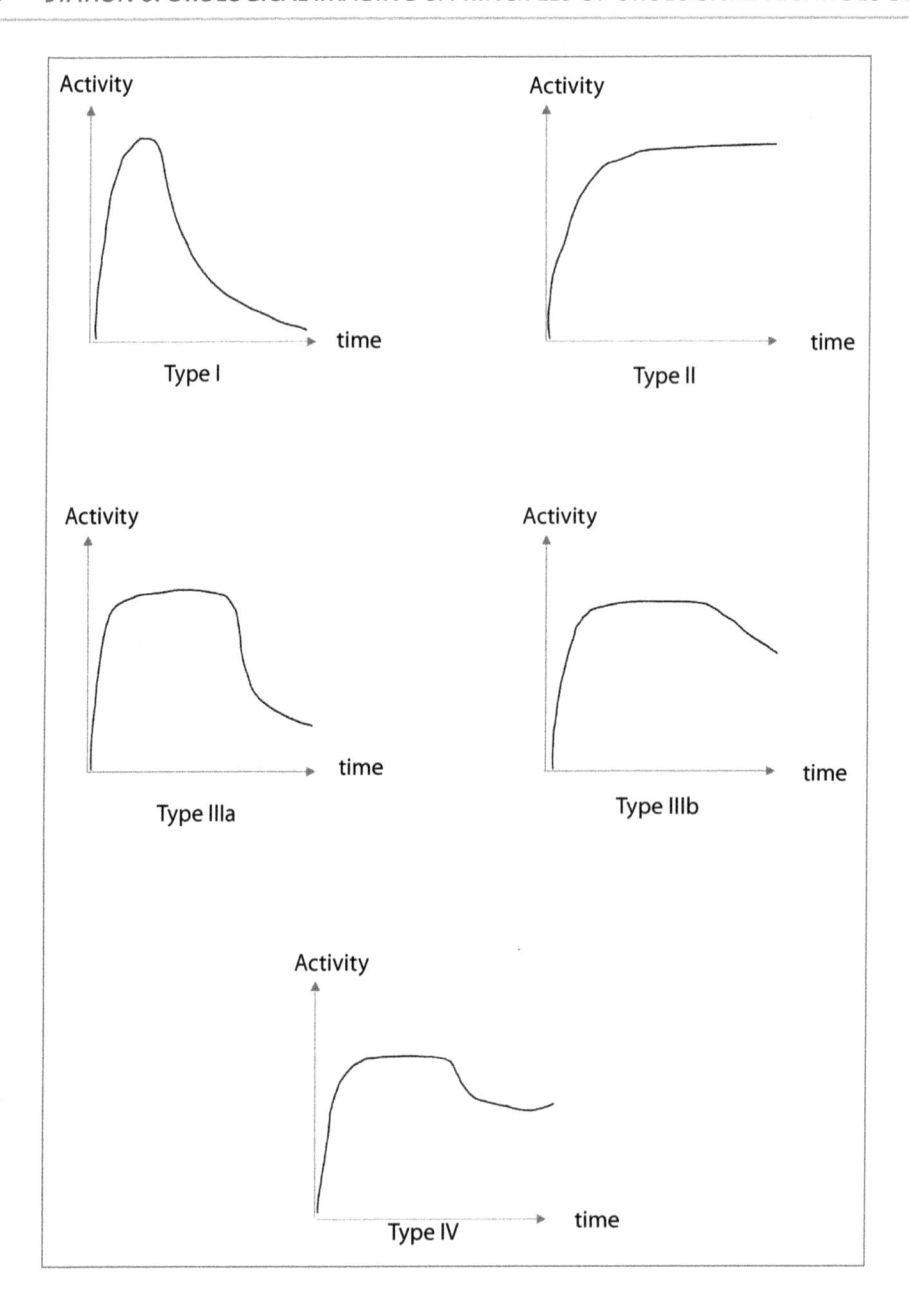

Figure 1 – Diuresis renogram curves for F+20

Whitaker Test

The Whittaker test is a mostly academic investigation for equivocal ureteric obstruction (e.g. type IIIb curve) rarely performed in modern practice (F-20 phase could be tried first).

It is an invasive test requiring percutaneous access tube to the renal pelvis and a urethral catheter. [10]

Saline is infused at 10mL / min via renal pelvis and the pressure difference is measured on the manometers on the renal tube and urethral catheter: [11]

- pressure difference > 22cm H_2O = ureteric obstruction
- pressure difference 15–22 cm H_2O = equivocal
- pressure difference < 15cm H_2O = obstructed

DMSA SCAN

DMSA scan is a static nuclear medicine study – producing a still image.

DMSA is a protein actively extracted and bound by functioning renal tubules, very little is filtered and it is not secreted.

The detail and resolution of the kidney produced in DMSA scans are much better than those of MAG3, for example showing cortical defects in acute pyelonephritis or scarring.

DMSA also gives good detail in duplex kidneys showing function of each moiety.

DMSA is most useful therefore where detailed information is required about the kidney and there is no concern for obstruction.

Infection may give a false reading – wait ≥ 6 weeks after resolution of infection before scanning.

RADIOISOTOPE

^{99m}Tc DMSA is a gamma-emitting radiopharmaceutical that binds to proximal convoluted tubule.

After injection DMSA accumulates slowly in the renal cortex – only a small amount is excreted in urine.

DMSA TECHNIQUE

The patient must wait 2–4 hours after DMSA injection to allow time for sufficient cortical uptake for any imaging to be undertaken.

Patient is then positioned supine on couch.

Static views of kidney are taken from different projections (e.g. anterior, posterior, oblique).

PET SCAN

PET is a form of nuclear medicine imaging which uses positron-emitting radionuclides rather than the gamma-emitting radionuclides used in renography.

There are several radionuclides suitable for PET – choice will depend on half-life of agent.

Most common radiotracer used in clinical practice is ^{18}F-labelled FDG:

- analogue of glucose
- more glucose required by anaerobic glycolysis in tumours than aerobic in normal tissue
- pronounced FDG uptake seen within tumours

FDG uptake is not specific to glucose metabolism within tumours.

FDG raised in areas of infection / inflammation, due to accumulation in macrophages / neutrophils

Choline (^{11}C) is recommended as the tracer for prostate cancer (less of it is excreted in the urine).

PET TECHNIQUE

The radiotracer is injected into patient and processed by body accumulating in tissue of interest.

When the tracer decays it emits a positron which should annihilate with a nearby electron to produce two back-to-back photons.

This encounter occurs along "line of response" – millions of these are recorded in typical PET scan and reconstructed to map out 3D distribution of radionuclide within body.

PET is often combined with CT allowing for information on tissue function from PET to be overlaid on structural information from the CT.

UROLOGICAL APPLICATIONS

For prostate cancer – to investigate biochemical relapse after RP or RTx (^{11}C)

Testicular cancer – for persisting nodal mass > 3cm in seminomatous GCT, (^{18}FDG)

Penile cancer – for assessment of nodal disease in advanced cases

FDG is not used in urothelial cancers as it is excreted by kidneys and accumulates in urinary tract.

PSMA scan is labelled with gallium (^{68}Ga) and is more expensive than standard ^{11}C PET as the radioisotope is less stable and cannot be stored.

PSMA has a higher sensitivity – EAU (2020) recommends this be offered to men with persistent PSA > 0.2ng / mL after radical treatment. [7]

SINGLE-PHOTON EMISSION COMPUTED TOMOGRAPHY

SPECT is similar to conventional PET except SPECT measures gamma radiation emitted directly (whereas PET measures positrons that have annihilated electrons nearby, emitting photons).

SPECT relies on radioisotope (e.g. Gallium) attached to a specific ligand, whose properties bind it to a certain type of tissue.

Gamma camera rotates around patient collecting images which are reconstructed to form a 3D image.

RADIOISOTOPE MEASUREMENT OF GFR

GFR can be measured by the blood clearance of any tracer that is cleared through the kidneys solely by glomerular filtration.

Nuclear medicine is ideal because it uses minute tracer quantities of radioisotope that do not disturb kidney function and give a very low radiation dose.

The method involves blood sampling alone and so is helpful when urine collection is difficult.

More reliable than creatinine clearance which requires 24-hour urine collection.

More accurate than eGFR which is based on a serum creatinine measurement in isolation.

Radioisotope measurement only gives total renal clearance, and so individual differential kidney clearance can be inferred in combination with either a MAG3 or DMSA.

^{51}Cr EDTA or ^{99m}Tc DTPA are options (solely cleared by glomerular filtration).

STUDY TECHNIQUE [12]

Patient is injected with selected radioisotope.

Blood samples are taken from opposite arm at 2, 3, 4 and 5 hours after injection.

These are then centrifuged to yield plasma which is then measured for radioactivity. A graph is plotted of plasma counts against time since injection.

The line is extrapolated back to time zero.

The slope determines the clearance rate.

NUCLEAR BONE SCAN

A nuclear medicine bone scan is a useful test for detecting areas of abnormal bone metabolism.

Indicated for identifying bone metastases presence and progression

^{99m}Tc MDP or ^{99m}Tc HDP are used.

They will show areas of normal and abnormal metabolism and are very sensitive.

They are also excreted in the urine, so kidney and bladder will also be seen on the image (i.e. hydronephrosis or urinary retention may be incidentally noted).

Typical radiation dose is 4–6mSv.

Three hours after injection, images showing bone metabolism are acquired in a variety of ways:

- whole body image: camera slowly moves along length of patient taking about 20 minutes to produce a whole-body scan,
- SPECT: the gamma camera rotates all the way round the patient taking images from many angles (20 minutes) which are then reconstructed

The bone scan has 3 phases:
- flow phase: within 60 seconds
- blood pool phase: within 5 minutes
- delayed phase: 2–4 hours

Areas of increased uptake, "hot spots," indicate increased bone metabolism.

These are not specific to metastases and may be seen in fractures, Paget's, and degeneration.

A "superscan" implies such diffuse bony metastatic infiltration that soft tissue / kidney / bladder uptake is reduced.

OPTICS, SCOPES AND ACCESSORIES

HOPKINS ROD-LENS SYSTEM

This involves a series of long glass rods in a metal cylinder separated by short airspaces.

Light is transmitted by optic fibre bundles running from external light source (usually halogen light which is yellow, hence the need for white balancing).

The advantages of the Hopkins Rod-Lens system include:
- superior light passage and image quality
- reduced diameter of instrument
- colour reproduction

This particular type of lens is only used in rigid cystoscopes.

OPTIC FIBRES

Optic fibres are flexible glass (or plastic) fibres that allow light to pass through them via a process called total internal reflection.

Fibres are grouped together in parallel fashion and protected by external plastic sleeves.

They are used for rigid / flexible URS.

Optic fibres within urology have two main uses:
- transmission of light from external source to endoscope: the fibres need not be coherent
- transmission of images: this relies on coherent bundles of optic fibres

The distal tip objective lens can be angled to give an oblique view – e.g. 12°, 30°, and 70°.

Digital scopes utilise a chip at the distal end of the scope which transmits a digital image.

SCOPES

The French Gauge (Fr) was developed by Charriere – corresponds to 3x the diameter (in mm).

For example a 21Fr cystoscope sheath has an external diameter of 7mm.

Semi-Rigid URS

Rigid scopes use fibre-optics for image transmission and not the rod-lens system.

The working element is approximately 34cm long.

The tip of the instrument is 7–10Fr.
- one working channel implies 3.4Fr
- if two channels are present, they are approximately 2.3Fr each

Flexible URS

Length may vary between 70–80cm.

Distal end of the instrument is 5.4Fr (working channels 3.6Fr approximately), which permit passage of instruments such as baskets or LASER fibre.

Flexible URS may be passed into kidney via access sheath.

Disposable scopes are digital, single-use and have no need for white-balancing.

Cystoscopes

Adult cystoscope sheaths are generally between 17–25Fr (approximately 30cm long).

These have a telescope inside, a bridge / working element and an outer sheath.

The telescope may be angled depending on the procedure:
- $0°$ marked as green
- $30°$ marked as red
- $70°$ marked as yellow

Resectoscopes are larger, usually 26–28Fr in size.

A leak test should be undertaken prior to use and before cleaning the scope – this is to check whether fluid is entering the scope.

Attach a manometer to the scope and inflate – the pressure should be maintained, if it is not this suggests a leak is present and the scope should be sent for repair.

Access Sheath

Access sheaths are used to establish a conduit during endourological procedures, to facilitate the repeated passage of instruments to the upper tract.

Access sheaths can be 40–45cm in length and 10–14Fr.

Access sheaths are hydrophilic (dampen before use), consist of an internal obturator and an outer sheath, lumen is made of PTFE, distal tip starts at 6Fr and tapers wider.

They decrease intra-renal pressure during URS.

ENDOSCOPIC INSTRUMENTS

Albarran bridge

Albarran lever / bridge is required for the endoscopic deflection of peripheral instruments.

You must ensure the level is flat to the scope when inserting this into urethra, otherwise the lever can injure the urethral lining and / or cause false passages.

Alligator and Biopsy Forceps

These have to be completely outside the working channel, otherwise the hinge mechanism will not be able to open properly.

Stone Cone

Device which can be deployed within the ureter, proximal to the stone, to prevent proximal migration of fragments during intra-corporeal lithotripsy

Nitinol inner core with PTFE outer layer

Baskets

There are many different baskets available for use in endourology.

Most have a straight tip guide, placed beyond the stone providing greater stability when in use.

The handles of all modern baskets can be dismantled to allow backward removal of the URS whilst basket remains in place.

This is invaluable when the basket and stone gets trapped in the ureter, permitting removal of the scope and re-insertion alongside the basket.

Wires

Guidewires in the ureter are placed for access, security and increasing stability of the ureter.

The diameter is 0.035in or 0.038in (typical length 150cm).

Important variable characteristics of wires include tip shape, shaft rigidity, torque (property that allows movement at one end to be transmitted to distal end) and surface resistance.

Guidewire selection depends on the circumstances demanded by the procedure.

Access to the ureter is often achieved via sensor wire:

- hydrophilic flexible tip (to minimise trauma) (tungsten filled for fluoroscopic visualisation)
- nitinol (nickel titanium alloy) / stainless steel core
- PTFE coating to offer smooth wire surface

Guidewires with higher rigidity are chosen when greater stability needed e.g. Amplatz super-stiff.

- large inner stainless-steel core
- PTFE coating for smoothness

When there is difficulty negotiating tortuous anatomy, a slippery hydrophilic guidewire is chosen, such as the Terumo® guidewire:

- nitinol core covered with polyurethane containing tungsten
- hydrophilic polymer coating

Ureteric Catheter

Approximately 6Fr in size, length 70cm, PTFE coated

Most have 1cm markings along the length.

STENTS AND CATHETERS

URETERIC STENTS

Most urine drains around stent by coaptive peristalsis rather than through central lumen, except at points of complete obstruction where it passes through side holes into the lumen.

Different materials can be used to make stents; most of these are polymers.

The presence of silicone increases rigidity and allows a lifetime of ≤ 12 months.

Implanted plastic tubes will cause production of sialomucins dependent upon their composition.

All tubes in the urinary tract will develop a biofilm and become encrusted with constituents of the urine, and will encrust more rapidly in stone-former's urine.

Foreign bodies should remain in situ for shortest time possible in stone formers, as encrustation starts within days of implantation and may occlude the stent lumen within a week.

All plastic stents require insertion over a guidewire under radiological control.

The whole length of a double J stent has small holes drilled in them to facilitate drainage.

Double J stents are between 18–30cm long (preformed coil at each end) and 4.7–8Fr.

Stents may be coated with hydrophilic Teflon or antibacterial coatings to make insertion easier or to try and reduce bacterial adherence and encrustation.

Radio-opacity of stents is increased by coating them with metals such as bismuth and barium.

INDICATIONS FOR STENTING

The indications for stent insertion can be divided into elective vs. emergency.

Emergency indications include:
- relief of ureteric obstruction
- trauma to the ureter
- drainage of acutely infected kidney

Elective indications include:
- protection of anastomosis (e.g. pyeloplasty, ureteric reimplantation)
- pre-operatively to aid identification of the ureter
- to protect drainage in endo-urological stone procedures

METALLIC STENT

Metallic ureteric stents are used mainly in management of ureteric strictures.

The *Memokath* stent is made of Nitinol (nickel-titanium memory shape alloy).

They are not widely used in clinical practice and pose challenges such as encrustation and difficulty when requiring replacement.

Resonance stents are made of metallic alloy, they can stay longer in-situ and are inserted through an 8Fr outer sheath.

MULTI-LENGTH STENT

Some stents have a multi-length coil on either end which means that the stent uncoils in capacious areas such as renal pelvis or bladder.

Main advantage is that fewer lengths of stent need to be kept in stock.

Polaris™ stents have a double-coil in bladder to reduce stent symptoms – not often used.

PROSTATIC / URETHRAL STENTS

These were developed to treat men with recurrent urethral strictures, BOO unfit for surgical intervention, or rarely for treating DetSD.

Almost all such stents have disappeared from the market.

Reasons for their lack of establishment in urological practice include:
- advances in anaesthesia and minimally invasive BOO surgery
- migration of stent resulting in urinary retention
- encrustation and blockage
- urinary tract infection
- incontinence (if striated urethral sphincter is held open)

URINARY CATHETERS

Urinary catheters are inserted for three main reasons:
- drainage of urine for diagnostic or therapeutic intent
- access to flush medications (e.g. BCG, MMC)
- diagnostic studies (e.g. urethrogram, cystogram)

The variables when describing a urethral catheter may include:
- *size*: expressed in French scale (Charriere gauge)
- *channels*: usually 2- or 3- way
- *tip design*: Foley (standard), Tiemann (curved tip), Coude (curved tip)
- *materials*: silicone (long-term ≤ 3 months) or PTFE / latex (short-term ≤ 28 days)

Catheter ring colours include 12F (white), 14F (green), 16F (orange), 18F (red).

Catheter by-passing can be managed with anticholinergics and reducing balloon size.

All patients will develop bacteriuria within 28 days – treat only if systemic symptoms, the catheter will have adherent bacteria called biofilm over it and will need replacing.

Antibiotic prophylaxis is not recommended to prevent catheter associated UTI.

There is a 5% daily rate of bacteriuria with an indwelling catheter.

If a catheter-related UTI is suspected, EAU (2020) recommends that the catheter should be replaced provided it has already been in-situ for ≥ 2 weeks. [13]

Biofilm Formation

A biofilm is a consortium of micro-organisms in which cells stick to each other and surface.

This confers a survival advantage to the microbes such that infections are resistant to antibiotics. [14]

There are 5 stages to biofilm formation:
1. adhesion to surface
2. aggregation
3. biofilm formation
4. 3-dimensional growth
5. micro-organism release to colonise other surfaces

LITHOTRIPSY

The components of ESWL include:

1. Energy source – can be electrohydraulic, electromagnetic, piezoelectric – the resulting shockwave that is produced is the same
2. Coupling mechanism – a gel or water-filled cushion is used to transmit the energy
3. Imaging – US or fluoroscopy can be used to localise the stone
4. Focusing system – required to concentrate energy on stone, elliptical (electrohydraulic ESWL), hemi-spherical (piezoelectric ESWL), cylindrical reflector (electromagnetic ESWL)

ELECTROHYDRAULIC ESWL

Electrohydraulic lithotripsy was one of the first methods of disrupting stones but is largely obsolete in clinical practice.

These produce a spark between two electrodes under water which results in rapid expansion and collapse of gas bubble and subsequent energy transmission. [Image 2]

This causes mechanical disintegration of stones into pieces that require extraction.

Electrohydraulic lithotripsy requires aqueous irritants (i.e. not saline or glycine).

It should not be used in the ureter as it may result in perforation (usually used for bladder stones).

ELECTROMAGNETIC ESWL

This relies on a cylindrical electromagnetic source – a coil of wire in close proximity to a thin metal membrane with water on the other side.

Current passes through the coil which repulses the metal membrane and generates a pressure pulse in water – this is focused by an acoustic lens. [Image 2]

This is the most common type of ESWL used currently.

PIEZOELECTRIC ESWL

Piezoelectric materials consist of ceramic or crystal elements that produce an electrical discharge under stress or tension.

Energy transmission is produced via movement of the source when electricity is passed through it.

Piezoelectric elements are placed on a concave surface which focuses the waves onto the stone. [Image 2]

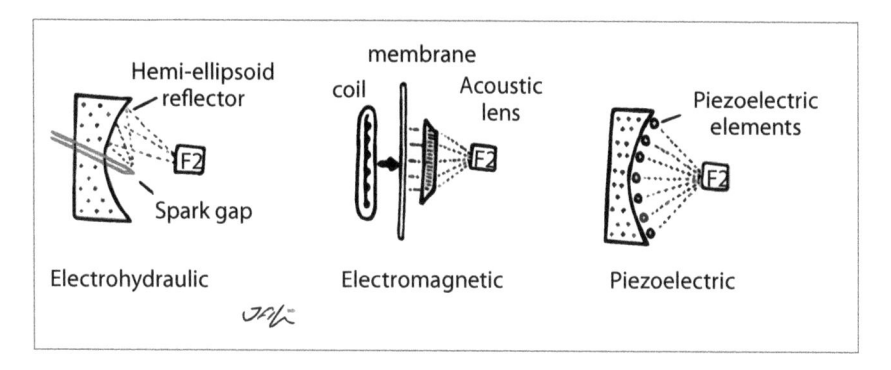

Image 2 – Diagrammatic representation of the 3 types of ESWL

INTRA-CORPOREAL LITHOTRIPSY

Ultrasonic Lithotripsy

The US waves produced by a generator are transmitted down a hollow probe resulting in vibration of the probe tip, which in contact with stone causes drilling and breakage.

Not for use in ureter as tip vibration causes heat production which may result in perforation.

Ballistic Lithotripsy

Forward momentum of metal rod placed in contact with stone surface

Swiss LithoClast™ uses a controlled burst of compressed air to move a projectile. Has tendency to move stones forward and can only be used in rigid scope.

Swiss LithoClast™ Master combines US with ballistic and suction. Often used in PCNL, however not in the ureter as the hot US tip may cause injury.

SHOCK-WAVE PHASES

The acoustic shockwave has two main phases:

- firstly, a short positive phase, causing erosion and entry and exit points of the stone, and internal shattering due to compressive effects of the wave
- secondly, a longer negative pressure phase which results in formation of microbubbles, which collapse and form micro-jets which further erode the stone

You may be asked in the FRCS (Urol) viva to draw the waveform. [Image 3]

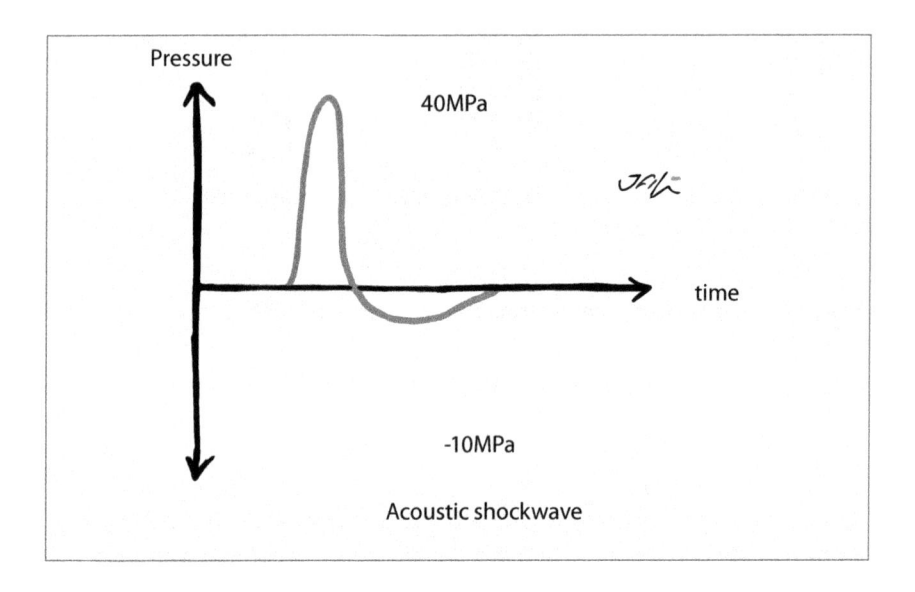

Image 3 – Waveform of shockwave

LASER LITHOTRIPSY

LASER is created by applying energy to a lasing medium, where a photon is released from an atom within the medium, and further collides with excited atoms to release more photons.

This process is called spontaneous emission.

The most commonly used LASER is the holmium: yttrium-aluminium-garnet (Ho:YAG).

Typical wavelength is 2140nm (invisible) (fibres are 200μm for kidney and 300μm for ureter).

LASER fibres are made of silica / silicon dioxide (i.e. glass).

Characteristics of LASER light include:

- *mono-chromatic* (single colour) defined by its wavelength
- *collimated* (travel in parallel beam) guided through optical fibres focused on small spot
- *coherent* (waves are in phase)

Tissue is affected by LASER energy by absorbing light and converting it to thermal energy.

It will target a tissue that absorbs the particular wavelength it is set at.

LASER energy breaks stones by:

- vaporisation – temperatures reach > 100°C
- photo-acoustic mechanism – whereby pulsed LASER forms plasma bubbles which expand and collapse generating a shockwave

LASER effects are limited to ≤ 1mm from fibre tip, hence risk of urothelial injury is minimised.

The different types and applications of LASERs within urology are shown in (Table 2).

Table 2 – LASERs used in urology and their properties [15]

Active Crystal	Abbreviation	Wavelength (nm)	Applications	Penetration (mm)
Holmium	Ho:YAG	2140	HoLEP, ablation of TCC Stone fragmentation	0.4
Neodynium	Nd:YAG	1064	Ablation of TCC Coagulation of prostate tissue	10
Kalium titanyl phosphate (Greenlight)	KTP:Nd:YAG	532	Absorbed by haemoglobin, used to vaporise prostate tissue	0.8
Lithium borate (Greenlight)	LBO:Nd:YAG	532	Absorbed by haemoglobin, used to vaporise prostate tissue	0.8
Thulium	Tm:YAG	2013	Ablation of TCC Vaporisation of prostate	0.25

LASER SAFETY

The main risks of LASER are burns and injuries to the eye.

Different LASERs pose different risks e.g. Nd:YAG has penetration depth of 10mm and can cause retinal injuries, whilst Ho:YAG may cause corneal injuries.

In the FRCS (Urol) viva you may be asked; "How do you make your theatre LASER-safe".

The following modifications should be implemented for the theatre set-up:

- signs outside the doors which should be locked
- minimise number of staff entering / exiting theatre
- safety goggles on all staff and patient
- LASER pedal should be protected to avoid inadvertent activation
- machine should be on standby at all times when not in use
- any clinician using the LASER should have up-to-date LASER safety training certificate
- windows should be blocked with curtains to prevent any reflection

THEATRE DESIGN, CLEANING AND EQUIPMENT

DEFINITIONS OF CLEANING

Sterilisation is the complete destruction of living organisms (including spores and viruses).

Disinfection removes most viable organisms but not necessarily some viruses and spores:

- most commonly using moist heat or liquid chemicals
- moist heat is safe and leaves no toxic residues, temperature typically 73–90°C
- chemical disinfectants are either alkylating or oxidising agents

Cleaning physically removes contamination but does not necessarily destroy micro-organisms:

- can take place in a washer at ≤ 35°C

Decontamination is a combination of processes that include cleaning, disinfection and/or sterilisation to render a medical device reusable and minimise risk transmission of infection.

AUTOCLAVING

Autoclaving is a process that combines heat and pressure to sterilise instruments (by combining pressure with heat, the temperature of water may be raised above boiling points).

Typical variables of autoclave are pressure, temperature and time.

A typical cycle would include 134°C for 3 minutes (or 121°C for 15 minutes).

Flexible scopes cannot withstand the conditions of autoclaving (rigid scopes can), and they require high level disinfection (soak time ≤ 30 minutes).

LEVELS OF DISINFECTION

These are divided into three classes according to the Spaulding Classification:

- *critical*, these penetrate tissue (require sterilisation before and after use)
- *semi-critical*, contact mucous membranes (e.g. cystoscopes)
- *non-critical*, only contact intact skin (e.g. blood pressure cuff)

THEATRE DESIGN

A key principle is the flow concept of a patient moving from outer "dirty" zone to clean zone between reception and theatre.

All used instruments and the patient should be moved back into the outer zone as soon as possible.

Prior to surgery, wherever possible the patient should be pre-assessed and the presence of infections (e.g. MRSA, COVID-19) should be treated before they go to theatre.

Patient should have showered and any hair local to incision removed if it interferes with operation.

Operative site should have gross contamination before antiseptic skin preparation, and the antiseptic agent should be applied in concentric circles out towards the periphery.

VENTILATION

Provided by vertical or horizontal laminar air flow with positive pressure air moving from the clean to the dirty environments.

Air goes through HEPA filters which remove particles > 0.3mm in diameter with an efficiency of 99.9%.

20–40 air changes / hour are normal but can be increased to 400 by a laminar flow hood.

An optimum temperature of 20–22°C and humidity of 50–55% should be set.

Warming blankets, bear-hugger, heating of IV and irrigation fluids are ways of maintaining patient's core temperature intra-operatively.

Air temperature in aseptic zone should be 1°C lower than clean zone to facilitate air movement.

THEATRE SAFETY

WHO Checklist

The WHO five steps to safe surgery include: [16]

1. team brief
2. sign in
3. time out
4. sign out
5. debrief

List Planning

In the FRCS (Urol) viva you may be given a list of patients with different needs and characteristics and be asked to devise the correct order of the list for the day.

1st – prioritise latex allergy, septic, pregnancy, children, diabetics

Last – infected cases

MRSA positive patients should be deferred, treated and relisted. If this is not possible then they should be placed last on the list.

Latex allergy

For patients with latex allergy, all staff must wear latex-free gloves.

The anaesthetic tubing must be latex-free and cleaned as gas can carry particles – therefore place first on the list or take a break after the preceding case to clean the tubing.

SUTURES

There are many variables when considering suture materials including:

- absorbable vs. non-absorbable
- mono- vs. poly-filaments (mono- has less tissue trauma but less memory)
- synthetic vs. natural

Choice will depend on the tissue being approximated and intention of the surgeon.

In closing abdominal wounds, a 4:1 ratio of suture to wound length is recommended.

In urology there is a risk of non-absorbable clips / sutures / staples coming into contact with urine and becoming a nidus for infection or stone formation.

Table 3 – Different types of sutures and their properties [17]

Generic name	Trade name	Characteristic	Absorption time	Use
Polyglactin	Vicryl	Synthetic, braided, absorbable	50–70 days	Tissue closure
Polyglactin	Vicryl rapide	Synthetic, braided, absorbable	40 days	Circumcision
Polydioxanone	PDS	Synthetic, monofilament, absorbable	180–210 days	Abdominal wound closure
Poliglecaprone	Monocryl	Synthetic, monofilament, absorbable	90–120 days	Tissue closure
Silk	Mersilk	Natural, braided, non-absorbable	N/A	Tissue closure
Polypropylene	Prolene	Synthetic, monofilament, non-absorbable	N/A	Vascular anastomoses

ENERGY IN SURGERY

Diathermy is the passage of high-frequency alternating current through body tissue, and where concentrated it can produce temperature $\leq 1000^\circ C$ to cut or coagulate tissues.

Standard electrical current would alternate at 60Hz.

At this frequency, current could be transmitted through body tissue but would result in excessive neuromuscular stimulation and possibly electrocution.

Nerve / muscle stimulation ceases at 100 kHz, so diathermy is safe above this frequency.

Tissue effects of diathermy:
- \> 45°C causes protein denaturation
- \> 90°C causes desiccation (sow) and vaporisation (fast)
- \> 200°C all tissues reduced to carbon

MONOPOLAR DIATHERMY

Monopolar diathermy involves the delivery of high-frequency current from a diathermy generator to the active electrode (e.g. forceps, resectoscope loop or ball).

Active electrode has small surface area (and therefore high current density) delivering heat at the point of tissue contact.

Current spreads from this point throughout the body returning to generator via patient electrode plate (Earth plate) which is the diathermy pad placed on the patient.

The pad has a large surface area (current density is low therefore minimal heat generated).

The pad should be placed on area of skin which is dry and hair-free for best contact.

BIPOLAR DIATHERMY

In bipolar diathermy the current passes down one limb of the forceps (active electrode) and back to the generator via the other limb (patient electrode plate).

There is no need for a patient pad to be placed.

Principle advantage is that current does not pass through body parts which are not being treated.

This allows greater precision about the quantity of tissue being coagulated (i.e. tissue next to the forceps will not be heated).

Only bipolar diathermy should be used for penile procedures such as circumcision.

If monopolar were used there would be the risk that all current passes through the common penile artery, thus eliminating the sole blood supply to the penis.

SAFETY

Although bipolar is inherently safer than monopolar, both come with potential risks:

- burns
- explosions (e.g. if inflammable anaesthetic agents are used)
- electrocution
- nerve injury / stimulation (e.g. obturator kick)
- end artery and tissue necrosis
- pacemakers

Burns can be avoided by ensuring adequate placement of patient plate, avoiding patient contact with metal objects (e.g. drip stand) and inflammable liquids (e.g. containing alcohol).

Pacemakers and Diathermy

Avoid all procedures with cardiac devices where possible.

If surgery is necessary, you must ensure surgical preparation involves:

- full device details including type, indication, date of implantation and last check
- careful consultation of cardiologist / pacemaker clinic / technician letters
- consider whether bipolar diathermy can be used alone

Implanted cardioverter defibrillators should be switched to "monitoring only" to avoid inadvertent activation (and switched back to normal function after surgery).

The following strategies can be used to increase safety in cardiac device settings:

- ensure diathermy plate placed such that current does not flow through device
- ensure optimal contact of diathermy plate
- avoid grounding via ECG leads
- use short bursts of diathermy only

CUTTING VS. COAGULATION

As the waveforms of the current change so do the corresponding tissue effects.

- "cut" waveform is high current and low voltage, producing heat very rapidly
- "coag" is a low intermittent waveform producing less heat so that a coagulum forms

Table 4 – Differences between cutting and coagulation diathermy [15]

Cutting	Coagulation
Continuous output (100% on)	Pulsed output (interrupted wave) (6% on)
Low voltage	High voltage
Intense heat (≤ 1000°C), more vaporisation	Less heat, more charring

HARMONIC SCALPEL

The harmonic instrument uses ultrasonic energy rather than electrical current as in diathermy.

US controls bleeding at lower temperature (< 100°C) by instrument blade vibrating at ≥ 50KHz, compressing vessel walls followed by sealing with coagulation of a protein coagulum.

This system minimises smoke generation, carbonisation of tissues and reduces potential damage to collateral structures.

LIGASURE

Ligasure uses a combination of pressure and continuous bipolar energy to create vessel fusion.

Radiofrequency melts collagen and elastin in vessel walls and reforms it into a permanent seal.

A feedback system automatically discontinues the energy delivery when the seal cycle is complete, preventing sticking or charring.

STATISTICS

Sensitivity	Proportion of patients who test positive among those who have the disease (rule in)
	No. of true positives / (No. of true positives + No. of false negatives)
Specificity	refers to test's ability to correctly reject healthy patients without a condition
	proportion of healthy patients known not to have disease, who test negative for it
	No. of true negatives / (No. of true negatives + No. of false positives)
PPV	Proportion with a positive test who actually have the disease
	PPV = No. of true positives / (No. of true positives + No. of false positives)
	Depends on how common the disease is in the study population
NPV –	Proportion with a negative test who do not have the disease
	NPV = No. of true negatives / (No. of true negatives + No. of false negatives)
Type 1 error	Inappropriate rejection of the null hypothesis
	indicates poor specificity (higher specificity yields lower type 1 error rate)
Type 2 error	Inappropriate acceptance of null hypothesis, often due to small numbers indicates poor sensitivity
Power	Probability of achieving a non-significant result when the null hypothesis is true
	Power ranges from 0 to 1 (as power increases, probability of making type 2 error of incorrectly failing to the reject the null decreases)
Absolute risk	Probability of an event in a particular group
	Number of events in group divided by number of people in that group

Relative risk Ratio of probability of outcome in exposed group to probability outcome in unexposed group (incidence exposed / incidence unexposed

        RR = 1 (exposure does not affect outcome)

        RR < 1 (risk of outcome is decreased by exposure)

        RR > 1 (risk of outcome is increased by exposure)

Odds ratio Ratio of odds of A in presence of B and the odds of A without presence of B

this statistic attempts to quantify the strength of association between A and B

NNT average number patients need to be treated to prevent one additional bad outcome

number needed to treat (NTT) is the reverse of ARR

NNT = 1 / ARR

Levels of Evidence

1a   Meta-analysis of RCTs

1b   At least one good RCT

2a   Well-designed, controlled experimental study

2b   Well-designed quasi-experimental study

3   Well-designed non-experimental study e.g case control series

4   Expert opinion

Grades of Recommendation

A Based on good quality studies, including at least one RCT

B Based on well-controlled clinical studies but no RCTs

C Made in the absence of directly applicable studies of good quality

MISCELLANEOUS

BLOOD PRODUCTS

A unit of packed red cells is 230–340mL and contains SAG-M (saline, adenine, glucose, mannitol) as the standard additive solution.

Donated blood is screened for HIV, hepatitis B / C, HIV.

Shelf-life ~ 35 days

Table 5 – Summary of ABO blood groups

Blood Group	Antigen on Cell	Antibodies in Plasma
O	None	Anti-A, anti-B
A	A	Anti-B
B	B	Anti-A
AB	AB	None

The complications of transfusion include:
- Early: allergic reaction, bruising, fever, acute haemolytic reaction
- Late: viral transmission

RENAL IMPAIRMENT

ACUTE KIDNEY INJURY

Acute kidney injury is classified by measuring the serum creatinine and determining the rise compared to the baseline reading.

Stage 1: 1.5–2x increase,

Stage 2: 2–3x,

Stage 3: > 3x

CHRONIC KIDNEY DISEASE

A patient can be diagnosed with CKD if they have abnormalities of kidney function or structure present for ≥ 3 months. [18]

CKD is classified based on the GFR (and level of proteinuria).

Table 6 – Classification of chronic kidney disease

GFR (mL / min)	Stage of CKD
≥ 90	1
60–89	2
45–59	3a
30–44	3b
15–29	4
< 15	5

DIALYSIS

Recall the indications for emergency dialysis – acidosis, electrolyte imbalance, intoxicants, overload, uraemia (mnemonic "AEIOU").

Haemofiltration is more likely to be used in the emergency / ITU setting.

Haemofiltration

Haemofiltration uses a highly permeable membrane.

Slow rate of blood flow (i.e. pump is not required), but a continuous process ongoing 24 hours / day from an artery and fed back into a vein.

Relies on hydrostatic pressure gradient across the membrane, removing solutes by filtration.

It will produce an ultrafiltrate and the movement of solutes is by convection.

Membrane has comparatively larger pores thus clearing more medium molecular weight solutes.

Haemodialysis

Blood is separated from dialysate by semi-permeable membrane.

Fast flow rate is required by pump to process large volumes of blood, as an intermittent process (e.g. 4-hour sessions, 3x / week).

Solute clearance is achieved by diffusion (speed depends on flow rate, osmotic pull, molecular size).

Cleaned blood is returned to the body and heparin is used to prevent clotting.

Peritoneal Dialysis

Peritoneal dialysis requires a surgical insertion of a peritoneal dialysis catheter (with risk of bowel injury and peritonitis).

Patient can flush 2–3L of dialysis fluid into the abdomen, using peritoneum as the membrane through which solutes and fluid are exchanged with blood.

After 4–6 hours the waste fluid is removed.

This process can be done continuously in "chronic ambulatory peritoneal dialysis."

Sclerosing peritonitis is a specific complication of peritoneal dialysis and involves bowel obstruction due to a thick fibrin layer within the peritoneum. [19]

Complications of Dialysis

Related to dialysis line – bleeding, pain, infection, clot / blockage, bacteraemia, endocarditis

Dis-equilibration syndrome – consequence of large volume fluid shifts (e.g. hypotension, fatigue)

Long-term sequalae – amyloidosis, cardiovascular disease, increased risk of renal cancer

Steal syndrome – ischaemia from reduced arterial flow distal to the fistula, causing hand pallor / necrosis / pain / reduced function, and may require ligation of the fistula [20]

HAEMOSTATIC AGENTS

There are many haemostatic agents used in surgery which can be based on collagen, cellulose, gelatin or polysaccharide spheres.

For the purpose of the FRCS (Urol) viva it is important to familiarise yourself with at least a couple of them, in case you are asked in the technology station.

Floseal® is a flowable white matrix that is packaged in a pre-filled syringe and works by:
- gelatin granules swell to produce tamponade effect
- high concentration of human thrombin converts fibrinogen to fibrin to form clot

Tachosil® – haemostatic agent in the form of a patch which is available in different sizes and works by:

- coated with fibrinogen and thrombin to promote coagulation cascade
- place on area with bleeding and apply gentle compression using a wet gauze

Surgicel® – a family of different products including powder, gauze haemostat and melting haemostat, which are all based on cellulose

IRRIGATION FLUIDS

The body's osmolarity is ~ 280–295mOsm / L.

Normal saline (isotonic) – contains 154mmol / L of Na+ and 154 mmol / L of Cl-.

1.5% glycine (hypotonic at 200mOsm / L) – is a non-ionic amino acid, used for monopolar surgery as it does not have free ions to carry charge from the electrode to the plate (saline has free ions).

NOVEL PROCEDURES FOR BLADDER OUTFLOW OBSTRUCTION

REZUM® PROCEDURE

The Rezum® device consist of a portable generator and a single-use disposable delivery device.

Radiofrequency energy is produced by the generator and applied to a conductive coil in the delivery device, producing thermal energy in the form of water vapour.

The steam is delivered to the transition zone of the prostate via a needle (penetration depth 10mm) to ablate the tissue and trigger cell necrosis.

Irrigation fluid of choice is normal saline.

UROLIFT PROCEDURE

UroLift® can be performed under local or general anaesthesia with antibiotics at induction.

The UroLift® system comprises of 2 single-use components – delivery device and implants (made of nitinol / stainless steel).

One end of the implant is anchored in the urethra and the other attached to the outer surface of the prostatic capsule – usually 4 are required.

Patients are safe to have an MRI scan after UroLift®.

Contraindications include – active UTI, visible haematuria, large median lobe, prostate > 100cc.

Migrated implants can lead to bladder stone formation.

L.I.F.T. Study

The L.I.F.T. study was originally a randomised single-blind study in men > 50 years, with IPSS > 12 and a prostate volume of 30–80cc. L.I.F.T study then followed up for 5 years. [21]

Patients underwent UroLift® (n = 140) and sham cystoscopy (n = 66).

Primary outcomes at 5 years included IPSS, QOL, Q_{max} and adverse events.

UroLift® was shown to improve IPSS by 88% and Q_{max} by 44% respectively.

PROSTATE ARTERY EMBOLISATION

PAE usually used the femoral artery as access to the prostatic arteries, which are embolized with polyvinyl alcohol (PVA).

PAE is approved by NICE (2018). [22]

UK ROPE Study [23]

A UK study designed to assess the efficacy and safety of PAE for LUTS due to BPH as well as conduct an indirect comparison of PAE with TURP

Primary outcome was improvement in IPSS and complication post-PAE.

Patients were recruited but not randomised to PAE (n = 216) and TURP (n = 89).

Study found that PAE was not as effective as TURP however it was safe and provided a statistically significant improvement in IPSS.

UROLOGICAL IMAGING AND PRINCIPLES OF UROLOGICAL TECHNOLOGY MCQS

1. Which of the following sutures is not absorbable?
   A) monocryl
   B) vicryl
   C) catgut
   D) polypropylene
   E) polydioxanone

2. How many times per hour is the air changed in the operating theatre in conventional ventilation systems?
   A) 20–40
   B) 40–60
   C) 60–80
   D) 80–100
   E) 100–120

3. What is the correct wavelength (nm) for KTP Greenlight LASER?
   A) 266
   B) 532
   C) 1064
   D) 2013
   E) 2140

4. What is the penetration depth (mm) of the Ho:YAG LASER?
   A) 0.1
   B) 0.2
   C) 0.4
   D) 0.8
   E) 10

5. What is the correct diameter (inches) for a typical guidewire in endourology?
   A) 0.035
   B) 0.048
   C) 0.125
   D) 0.148
   E) 0.152

6. Which parameter is not included as part of the MDRD formula for calculating GFR?
   A) age
   B) gender
   C) serum creatinine
   D) ethnicity
   E) body mass

7. What is the approximate half-life of ^{99m}Tc?
   A) 24 hours
   B) 18 hours
   C) 12 hours
   D) 9 hours
   E) 6 hours

8. Which radioisotope does the PMSA scan use?
   A) ^{11}C
   B) ^{68}Ga
   C) ^{131}I
   D) ^{99m}Tc
   E) ^{192}Ir

9. What is the correct external diameter (mm) of a 24Fr cystoscope?
   A) 24
   B) 16
   C) 12
   D) 8
   E) 6

UROLOGICAL IMAGING AND PRINCIPLES OF UROLOGICAL TECHNOLOGY MCQS

10. The nursing assistant passes you a cystoscope with a red label. What is the correct degree angle of this scope?
    A) 0
    B) 12
    C) 30
    D) 70
    E) none of the above

11. Ureteric stents are radiopaque – which metal / alloy do they contain which allows for this property?
    A) bismuth
    B) iron
    C) steel
    D) nickel
    E) titanium

12. What gauge (Fr) is a urinary catheter with an orange coloured label?
    A) 12
    B) 14
    C) 16
    D) 18
    E) 20

13. Which of the following is not a recognised stage of biofilm formation?
    A) aggregation
    B) adhesion
    C) 3D growth
    D) replication
    E) microorganism release

14. During ESWL, what is the approximate pressure value at the top of positive phase waveform of the acoustic shockwave?
    A) 10MPa
    B) 40Mpa
    C) 10KPa
    D) 40KPa
    E) 80Kpa

STATION 6: UROLOGICAL IMAGING & PRINCIPLES OF UROLOGICAL TECHNOLOGY

15. What type of energy does the harmonic scalpel use?
    A) Monopolar
    B) Bipolar
    C) Thermal
    D) Radiofrequency
    E) Ultrasound

16. What level of evidence is a well-designed, controlled experimental study?
    A) 1a
    B) 1b
    C) 2a
    D) 2b
    E) 3

17. What is the correct osmolarity (mOsm / L) for 1.5% glycine solution?
    A) 200
    B) 220
    C) 230
    D) 250
    E) 280

18. What type of energy dose the ligasure device use?
    A) Monopolar
    B) Bipolar
    C) Thermal
    D) Radiofrequency
    E) Ultrasound

19. What are LASER fibres made of?
    A) nitinol
    B) silica
    C) PTFE
    D) carbon
    E) titanium

20. What is the correct wavelength (nm) for Ho:YAG LASER?
    A) 266
    B) 532
    C) 1064
    D) 2013
    E) 2140

REFERENCES

1. Napier-Hemy R. (2012) Principles of Measurement of Urinary Flow. In: Payne S, Eardley I, O'Flynn K, Imaging and Technology in Urology, Springer-Verlag, London.
2. Allisy-Roberts PJ. (2005) Radiation quantities and units—understanding the sievert. *Journal of Radiological Protection*, 25(1), 97.
3. Little MP, Wakeford R, Tawn EJ, et al. (2009) Risks associated with low doses and low dose rates of ionizing radiation: why linearity may be (almost) the best we can do. *Radiology*, 251(1), 6–12.
4. American College of Radiology – Manual on Contrast Media. (2020) Available at: https://www.acr.org/-/media/ACR/Files/Clinical-Resources/Contrast_Media.pdf [last accessed 13 June 2020].
5. Royal College of Radiology – Standards for intravascular contrast administration to adult patients, 3rd edition. Available at: https://www.rcr.ac.uk/sites/default/files/Intravasc_contrast_web.pdf [last accessed 13 June 2020].
6. Grobner T, Prischl FC. (2007) Gadolinium and nephrogenic systemic fibrosis. *Kidney international*, 72(3), 260–264.
7. Mottet N, Cornford P, van den Bergh RCN, et al. (2020) EAU Guidelines: Prostate Cancer. Available at: https://uroweb.org/guideline/prostate-cancer/#6_2 [last accessed 13 June 2020].
8. Ahmed HU, Zacharakis E, Dudderidge T, et al. (2009) High-intensity-focused ultrasound in the treatment of primary prostate cancer: the first UK series. *British journal of cancer*, 101(1), 19–26.
9. Fritzberg AR, Abrams PG, Beaumier PL, et al. (1988). Specific and stable labeling of antibodies with technetium-99m with a diamide dithiolate chelating agent. *Proceedings of the National Academy of Sciences*, 85(11), 4025–4029.
10. Jaffe RB, Middleton Jr AW. (1980) Whitaker test: differentiation of obstructive from nonobstructive uropathy. *American Journal of Roentgenology*, 134(1), 9–15.
11. Lupton EW, George NJ. (2010). The Whitaker test: 35 years on. *BJU international*, 105(1), 94–100.
12. Lawson R. (2012) How to Do a Radioisotope Glomerular Filtration Rate Study. In: Payne S, Eardley I, O'Flynn K, Imaging and Technology in Urology, Springer-Verlag, London.
13. Bonkat G, Bartoletti R, Bruyere F, et al. (2020) EAU Guidelines: Urological Infections. Available at: https://uroweb.org/guideline/urological-infections/ [last accessed 14 June 2020].

14. Niveditha S, Pramodhini S, Umadevi S, et al. (2012) The isolation and the biofilm formation of uropathogens in the patients with catheter associated urinary tract infections (UTIs). *Journal of clinical and diagnostic research: JCDR, 6*(9), 1478.
15. Ellis G, Cohen D, Bycroft JA, et al. (2018) Urotechnology, Principles of Uroradiology and Miscellaneous. In: Arya M, Shergull IS, Fernando HS et al. Viva Practice for the FRCS (Urol) and Postgraduate Urology Examinations 2nd Edition, CRC Press, London.
16. Vickers R. (2011) Five steps to safer surgery. *The Annals of The Royal College of Surgeons of England, 93*(7), 501–503.
17. Fawcett D. (2012) Sutures and Clips. In: Payne S, Eardley I, O'Flynn K, Imaging and Technology in Urology, Springer-Verlag, London.
18. CKD stages. The Renal Association. Available at: https://renal.org/information-resources/the-uk-eckd-guide/ckd-stages/ [last accessed 14 June 2020].
19. Rigby RJ, Hawley CM. (1998) Sclerosing peritonitis: the experience in Australia. *Nephrology Dialysis Transplantation, 13*(1), 154–159.
20. Wixon CL, Hughes JD, Mills JL. (2000) Understanding strategies for the treatment of ischemic steal syndrome after hemodialysis access. *Journal of the American College of Surgeons, 191*(3), 301–310.
21. Roehrborn CG, Barkin J, Gange SN, et al. et al. (2017) Five year results of the prospective randomized controlled prostatic urethral LIFT study. *The Canadian journal of urology, 24*(3), 8802–8813.
22. NICE Guidelines (2018) Prostate artery embolization for lower urinary tract symptoms caused by benign prostatic hyperplasia. Available at: https://www.nice.org.uk/guidance/ipg611/chapter/1-Recommendations [last accessed 14 June 2020].
23. Ray AF, Powell J, Speakman MJ, et al. (2018) Efficacy and safety of prostate artery embolization for benign prostatic hyperplasia: an observational study and propensity-matched comparison with transurethral resection of the prostate (the UK-ROPE study). *BJU international, 122*(2), 270–282.

STATION 7
BLADDER DYSFUNCTION AND GYNAECOLOGICAL ASPECTS OF UROLOGY

URINARY TRACT INNERVATION

OVERACTIVE BLADDER

STRESS INCONTINENCE

POST-PROSTATECTOMY INCONTINENCE

URODYNAMICS

FEMALE URETHRAL DIVERTICULUM

FEMALE URINARY TRACT FISTULAE

PELVIC ORGAN PROLAPSE

CONTENTS

URINARY TRACT INNERVATION — 165
  BLADDER MOTOR INNERVATION — 165
  BLADDER SENSORY INNERVATION — 166
  URETHRAL SPHINCTER INNERVATION — 167
  MICTURITION CYCLE — 167
    FILLING PHASE — 167
    VOIDING PHASE — 168
  UROLOGICAL CHARACTERISTICS OF NEUROLOGICAL INJURIES — 169
    SUPRA-PONTINE LESIONS — 170
    SUPRA-SACRAL SPINAL CORD INJURIES — 170
    CAUDA EQUINA / CONUS (S1–5) / PERIPHERAL NERVE LESIONS — 170
    OTHER NEUROLOGICAL CONDITIONS — 170
  AUTONOMIC DYSREFLEXIA — 171

OVERACTIVE BLADDER — 173
  DEFINITIONS — 173
  EPIDEMIOLOGY — 173
  RISK FACTORS — 173
  DIAGNOSTIC EVALUATION — 174
    PATIENT HISTORY — 174
    PATIENT EXAMINATION — 176
    INVESTIGATIONS — 177
  MANAGEMENT — 178
    CONSERVATIVE MEASURES — 178
    BLADDER RETRAINING — 179
    PELVIC FLOOR MUSCLE TRAINING — 179
    ANTICHOLINERGICS — 179
    MIRABEGRON — 181
    VAGINAL OESTROGEN TREATMENT — 182
    BOTULINUM TOXIN — 183
    POSTERIOR TIBIAL NERVE STIMULATION — 185
    SACRAL NEUROMODULATION — 185
    CLAM AUGMENTATION CYSTOPLASTY — 186

STATION 7: BLADDER DYSFUNCTION AND GYNAECOLOGICAL ASPECTS OF UROLOGY

STRESS INCONTINENCE	**189**
DIAGNOSTIC EVALUATION	189
PATIENT HISTORY	189
PATIENT EXAMINATION	189
INVESTIGATIONS	190
MANAGEMENT	191
CONSERVATIVE MEASURES	191
DULOXETINE	191
BULKING AGENTS	192
MID-URETHRAL SLINGS	193
POST-PROSTATECTOMY INCONTINENCE	**197**
DIAGNOSTIC EVALUATION	197
PATIENT HISTORY	197
PATIENT EXAMINATION	197
MANAGEMENT	197
MALE SLINGS	198
ARTIFICIAL URETHRAL SPHINCTER	198
URODYNAMICS	**200**
DEFINITIONS	200
INDICATIONS	200
TECHNIQUE	201
DETRUSOR SPHINCTER DYSSYNERGIA	205
FEMALE URETHRAL DIVERTICULUM	**207**
AETIOLOGY	207
DIAGNOSTIC EVALUATION	207
PATIENT HISTORY	207
PATIENT EXAMINATION	207
IMAGING	208
CYSTOSCOPY	208
MANAGEMENT	208
FEMALE URINARY TRACT FISTULAE	**209**
VESICOVAGINAL FISTULAE	209
COLOVESICAL FISTULAE	209

VESICOUTERINE FISTULAE	209
PELVIC ORGAN PROLAPSE	**210**
AETIOLOGY	210
CLASSIFICATION	210
DIAGNOSTIC EVALUATION	211
PATIENT HISTORY	211
PATIENT EXAMINATION	211
MANAGEMENT	212
CONSERVATIVE	212
SURGICAL	212
BLADDER DYSFUNCTION AND GYNAECOLOGICAL ASPECTS OF UROLOGY MCQS	**213**
REFERENCES	**218**

URINARY TRACT INNERVATION

BLADDER MOTOR INNERVATION

LUT receives both sympathetic and parasympathetic innervation from the autonomic nervous system.

LUT also receives nerves from the somatic nervous system.

Parasympathetic

Pre-ganglionic fibres located in S2–4 spinal segments [1]

- → synapse with post-ganglionic fibres within detrusor muscle
- → provide excitatory input to bladder smooth muscle to cause detrusor contraction (i.e. motor)
- → provide inhibitory input to bladder neck / urethra (causing relaxation)

Sacral micturition centre (parasympathetic) stimulates detrusor contraction.

Sympathetic

Sympathetic cell bodies are located in spinal segments T10 – T12 and L1 – L2.

Innervate trigone, blood vessels of bladder, smooth muscle of prostate

Pre-ganglionic fibres synapse with post-ganglionic fibres in the hypogastric plexus

- → main function is inhibition of parasympathetic pathways (i.e. inhibiting contraction)
- → provides contraction of outflow tract (stimulates contraction of pre-prostatic sphincter)

Somatic

The somatic nerve to the pelvic floor musculature and external urethral rhabdosphincter (skeletal muscle) originates from S2–4 and is conveyed via the pudendal nerve.

The cells bodies lie in a distinct motor nucleus at same spinal level, called *Onuf's nucleus*, in the ventral part of the anterior horn of the sacral spinal cord. [2]

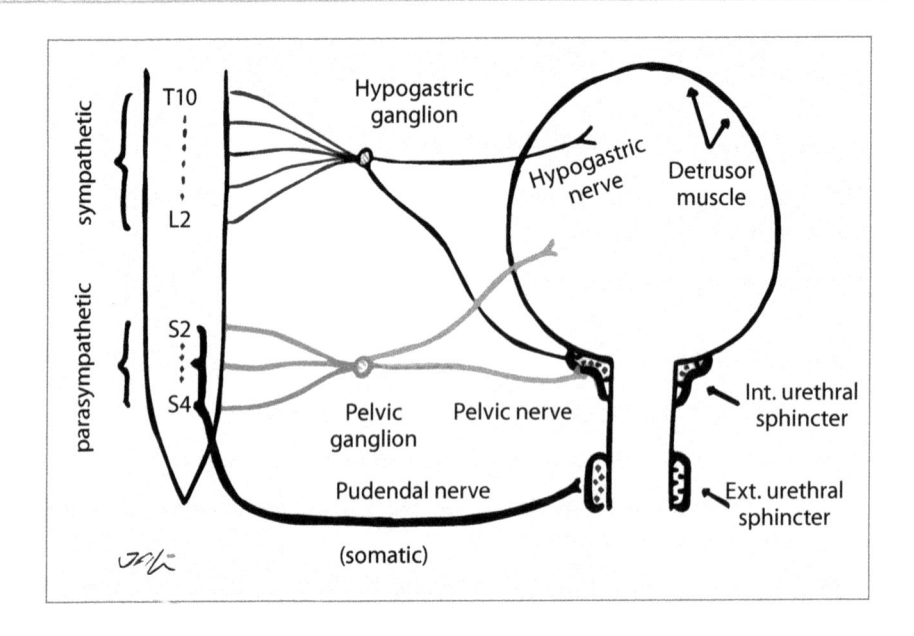

Image 1 – Motor supply to the bladder

BLADDER SENSORY INNERVATION

There are receptors throughout the bladder feeding afferent nerves, located in both detrusor muscle and sub-urothelial layer. [1]

Sensations of bladder fullness are conveyed to spinal cord in pelvic and hypogastric nerves.

Afferent nerves contain myelinated (Aδ) (respond to distension / contraction and filling information) and unmyelinated (C) fibres which respond to irritative stimuli and temperature.

Cell bodies located in dorsal root ganglia at S2–3 and T11 – L2

- → afferents enter spinal cord through dorsal horn
- → ascend to pontine micturition centre and cortex (via spinothalamic tracts)

Afferent fibres from trigone

- → run in hypogastric nerve and ascend thoracolumbar cord to pons / cerebral cortex

Afferent fibres from urethra

- run in pudendal nerve and ascend thoracolumbar cord to pons / cerebral cortex

The bulbocavernous (or bulbospongiosus) reflex checks the S2–4 arc: by squeezing the glans / clitoris or pulling on a urinary catheter, this should result in anal sphincter contraction.

URETHRAL SPHINCTER INNERVATION

The external urethral sphincter mechanism is distal to the apex of the prostate (between verumontanum and proximal bulbar urethra).

The external urethral sphincter has 3 components: [3]

1. *Extrinsic skeletal muscle*

   Outermost layer, pubo-urethral sling (part of levator ani), made of striated muscle innervated by pudendal nerve (S2–4 somatic), augments urethral occlusion pressure

2. *Smooth muscle within urethral wall*

   Cholinergic innervation for tone, relaxed by nitric oxide

3. *Intrinsic striated muscle*

   U-shaped skeletal muscle within the wall of the urethra (rhabdosphincter) – absent posteriorly, produces occlusion by kinking rather than circumferential compression.

Pre-ganglionic somatic nerve fibres derived from S2–4 (Onuf's nucleus)

→ travel to rhabdosphincter via perineal branch of pudendal nerve for motor input

→ active nerves contract sphincter / inhibit micturition

There is also input from pelvic plexus branches (i.e. not solely dependent on pelvic nerve).

MICTURITION CYCLE

FILLING PHASE

~98% of the micturition cycle is spent in the filling phase.

During bladder filling, the bladder pressure remains low. Recall that jeopardy of the upper tracts may occur if bladder pressures > 40cm H_2O.

Due to compliance (δV / δP) – mediated by the vesico-elastic properties of the bladder.

The bladder contains elastin and collagen fibres, as well as the ability of detrusor smooth muscle cells to increase in length without significant increase in tension.

Chronic obstruction / distension / raised pressure leads to fibrotic changes and stiffening.

As bladder fills, afferent activity from stretch receptors passes to pons and cerebral cortex.

In storage, when voiding is not to be initiated: [3]

- increased activity within external urethral sphincter
- central inhibition to decrease parasympathetic activity to detrusor
- "gating mechanism" within parasympathetic ganglia, whereby pre-ganglionic inhibit afferent activity via interneurons

Guarding reflex is gradual increase in striated sphincter activity by increased pudendal nerve activity during normal filling, to match the rising urethral pressure. [4]

VOIDING PHASE

Micturition should be initiated when appropriate.

Stretch receptors in bladder sense increasing tension, which is relayed via afferent neurons to the dorsal horn of sacral cord and conveyed to periaqueductal grey matter.

Periaqueductal grey is informed about bladder filling.

Periaqueductal grey (along with input from other brain area) feed pontine micturition centre to determine whether it is appropriate to void.

If micturition is appropriate, it is co-ordinated by Barrington's nucleus in the pontine micturition centre:

- EUS relaxation by somatic nerve inhibition in Onuf's nucleus
- followed by detrusor muscle contraction (S2–4 parasympathetic)

In supra-sacral SCI the patient thus risks developing DetSD.

UROLOGICAL CHARACTERISTICS OF NEUROLOGICAL INJURIES

Many neurological conditions are associated with abnormal bladder and sphincter function, and their symptomatology is defined as "neuropathic".

The bladder / sphincter may be over- or under- active and any combination may co-exist.

The normal observation should be a synergistic relationship:
- during filling, detrusor muscle is inactive and sphincter pressure is high
- during voiding, sphincter relaxes before and then detrusor muscle contracts

The main situation to avoid is a high-pressure system which may damage the upper tracts.

High Pressure Bladder – High Pressure Sphincter [5]

An overactive bladder in the neuropathic context is defined as detrusor hyperreflexia.

At times high bladder pressure overcomes the sphincter pressure and patient leaks urine, however the kidneys work against this system and thus develop hydronephrosis and eventual failure.

When sphincter pressure > bladder pressure, emptying is ineffective and patient may develop urinary retention, rUTI

An overactive sphincter generates high pressure during filling and voiding, and this is termed detrusor sphincter dyssynergia (DetSD).

Low Pressure Bladder – High Pressure Sphincter [5]

An underactive bladder in the neuropathic context is defined as detrusor areflexia.

Bladder will simply fill up and may not empty at all.

High Pressure Bladder – Low Pressure Sphincter [5]

Bladder only able to hold low volumes of urine before leaking (incontinence)

Low Pressure Bladder – Low Pressure Sphincter [5]

Detrusor areflexia may make patient dry most of the time.

Urine leakage may occur however in the context of raised abdominal pressure (sphincter incompetent), for example during transfer from wheelchair.

SUPRA-PONTINE LESIONS

For example in CVA or Parkinson's disease

Micturition reflexes are intact; however leakage may occur at inappropriate times due to DO, however pattern is normal and bladder pressures are safe

SUPRA-SACRAL SPINAL CORD INJURIES

These are lesions between the pons and L5 (i.e. between pontine micturition centre and sacral micturition centre).

Feature neurogenic DO, DetSD and low-compliance bladders, which may result in potentially unsafe high-pressure systems.

In lesions above T6 patients may encounter AD emergency.

CAUDA EQUINA / CONUS (S1–5) / PERIPHERAL NERVE LESIONS

The pattern of injury yields a lower motor neurone type of neurological pattern.

Characterised by areflexic bladder with urethral sphincter weakness (stress incontinence), generally with safer low-pressure systems

OTHER NEUROLOGICAL CONDITIONS

Multiple Sclerosis – most common issue is NDO, causing urgency / frequency symptoms.

Parkinson's disease – most common issue is NDO, patients tend to have acceptable sphincter function (i.e. no DetSD) and therefore voiding unobstructed (unless BOO). [6]
- patients tend to have poorer outcome after TURP surgery

Multiple System Atrophy (formerly Shy-Drager syndrome) – is a cause of Parkinsonism characterised by postural hypotension, the loss of pons cells causes detrusor hyperreflexia, the loss of Onuf's nucleus neurons denervates sphincter causing urinary incontinence. [7]

Spina bifida – is due to failure of fusion of neural and bony elements of the spine, hallmark UDS finding is loss of bladder compliance with increased outlet resistance (DetSD).

- mainstay of management is achieving low pressure system, continence and QOL improvement

AUTONOMIC DYSREFLEXIA

This is a potentially life-threatening medical emergency which occurs only in SCI patients.

AD may occur if lesion is above T6 (the sympathetic outflow) (i.e. more common in cervical lesions).

AD is a sudden and exaggerated autonomic (primarily sympathetic) response to various stimuli, which tend to be noxious and below the level of the SCI. [1]

Common stimuli that may lead to AD include: [8]

- bladder distension / irritation (most common – 75%)
- bowel distension / faecal impaction (2nd most common – 15%)
- iatrogenic urological interventions, UTI, urolithiasis
- non-urological causes can range from ingrown toenail to lower limb fractures

Pathogenesis

Noxious stimulus leads to sympathetic discharge – leading to reflex arterial vasoconstriction and therefore systemic hypertension.

Carotid bodies detect this rise in blood pressure and try to compensate with vagal reflex discharges which cause vasodilatation and bradycardia as homeostatic response.

This compensatory stimulus however cannot cross the level of the SCI injury.

Vasoconstriction and hypertension persists – below the level of injury the patient is pale and clammy, above the level of injury they are sweaty and flushed.

Diagnostic Evaluation

From the patient history the following should be elucidated:
- full details of SCI
- any previous episodes of AD
- screen for potential noxious stimuli

Patient examination should assess for:
- significant rise in systolic and diastolic blood pressure
- profuse sweating and flushing above the level of lesion, usually face / neck / shoulders
- pale clammy skin below level of lesion
- abdominal examination for palpable bladder / DRE for faecal impaction

Perform urinalysis (send MSU for culture if appropriate).

Perform bedside bladder scan, place patient on cardiac monitoring.

Management

The main principles of the management involve the following: [9]
- prompt recognition of the condition
- identification of precipitating factor and reversing this (e.g. catheter for retention)
- sit patient upright (induce orthostatic hypotension)
- administer sub-lingual glyceryl trinitrate and labetalol IV
- consider immediate release nifedipine
- close monitoring and early involvement of critical care outreach

Danger of AD is the hypertension which can lead to CVA, haemorrhage, convulsions and death.

Credé manoeuvre is a technique involving manual compression of the bladder (for patients with reduced bladder tone) and is most effective if low bladder outlet resistance, it is easier in children and slim adults however VUR is a relative contraindication.

OVERACTIVE BLADDER

DEFINITIONS

Overactive Bladder Syndrome is a symptom syndrome of:
- urgency with or without urge incontinence,
- usually accompanied with urinary frequency and nocturia,
- in the absence of pathological (e.g. stones, UTI) and metabolic factors (e.g. diabetes)

Idiopathic detrusor overactivity is a UDS diagnosis of evidence of detrusor contraction which may be spontaneous or provoked.

Urinary incontinence is the involuntary leakage of urine.

Urge urinary incontinence, involuntary leakage of urine preceded by urinary urgency

Stress urinary incontinence, involuntary leakage of urine on effort / exertion

Mixed urinary incontinence, involuntary leakage of urine associated with urgency and exertion / effort

Overflow incontinence, leakage of urine when bladder is abnormally distended with large PVR

Urethral hypermobility, condition of excessive movement and instability of the female urethra due to weakened urogenital diaphragm

EPIDEMIOLOGY

Prevalence of urinary incontinence is twice as common in females vs. males.

17% of population > 40 years in Europe have symptoms of OAB.

Prevalence of OAB rises with increasing age.

For women the prevalence of SUI (50%), UUI (11%) and MUI (36%).

RISK FACTORS

General risk factors predisposing to urinary incontinence include:
- *gender* – females are at higher risk
- *race* – Caucasians higher risk than Afro-Caribbeans
- *neurological* – such as MS, CVA, Parkinson's disease

- *childbirth* – vaginal (forceps) delivery, increasing parity, pregnancy
- *pelvic surgery / radiotherapy*
- *diabetes*

General risk factors promoting urinary incontinence include:
- smoking / chronic cough
- obesity, poor mobility
- old age, cognitive defects
- urinary infections
- oestrogen deficiency

DIAGNOSTIC EVALUATION

PATIENT HISTORY

A thorough patient history is the first step in the assessment of all patients with urinary incontinence.

The main aims of the history include:
- categorising patient as UUI, SUI or MUI
- identifying predisposing and promoting risk factors [listed above]
- identifying any red flag symptoms

The following points should be elucidated from the patient history:
- duration and onset of symptoms
- exacerbating factors
- description of any episodes of urinary incontinence
- number of pads required daily / impact on QOL
- details on fluid intake
- past urological / neurological / surgical / obstetric history
- any concurrent bowel / sexual function
- red-flag symptoms (visible haematuria, bladder pain)

In your FRCS (Urol) viva you should state you would see the patient in a dedicated functional urology clinic in presence of continence nurse specialist.

Validated patient-completed questionnaires are helpful although to date there is no single questionnaire that fulfils all requirements for assessment of patients with incontinence.

In your FRCS (Urol) viva you should propose using the ICIQ-short form questionnaire in your patient assessment for urinary incontinence [Table 1]

Table 1 – ICIQ-UI Short form questionnaire for urinary incontinence [10]

1. Date of birth	
2. Gender	Female
	Male
3. How often do you leak urine?	0 – Never
	1 – once a week or less
	2 – 2–3x / week
	3 – about once a day
	4 – several times a day
	5 – all the time
4. How much urine do you usually leak?	0 – none
	2 – small amount
	4 – moderate amount
	6 – large amount
5. Overall, how much does leaking urine interfere with your everyday life?	0 1 2 3 4 5 6 7 8 9 10
	Not at all A great deal
ICIQ Score:	Sum of Q3, Q4, Q5. (0–21)
When does urine leak?	Never – urine does not leak
	Leaks before you can get to the toilet
(not included in score)	Leaks when you cough or sneeze
	Leaks when you are asleep
	Leaks when you are physically active / exercising
	Leaks when you have finished urinating and are dressed
	Leaks for no obvious reason
	Leaks all the time

FVC or bladder diaries may have been completed prior to clinic attendance.

Bladder diary records the type and volume of fluid intake, incontinence episode, number of used pads along with urinary frequency and voided volume.

FVC only records urine volume and frequency and incontinence episodes.

Nocturnal polyuria is diagnosed from a bladder diary by night-time urine volume (includes first morning void) and is diagnosed if ≥ 1/3 of the total urine volume over 24 hours is passed at night.

PATIENT EXAMINATION

All examinations should be performed in the presence of a chaperone.

Both Sexes

Examine the abdomen for palpable bladder, scars and organomegaly.

Neurological examination should include assessment of gait, lower limb function, perineal sensation and lower spine visualisation / palpation.

Consider DRE to evaluate for constipation, palpable masses and anal tone assessment.

Women

Bimanual examination will reveal any pelvic masses.

Pelvic examination in the supine position should be undertaken to identify:
- signs of vaginal atrophy / dryness associated with oestrogen deficiency
- pelvic organ prolapse [consider POPQ – discussed in "Pelvic Organ Prolapse" station]
- digital assessment of strength of pelvic floor muscle contraction (Oxford Grading System)

Pelvic examination in left lateral position with Sim's speculum should be undertaken to evaluate for cystocoele or rectocoele.

Cough stress test with sufficiently full bladder should identify presence of SUI.

(Modified) Oxford Grading System

Tool developed to evaluate strength of pelvic floor muscles via a six-point scale (Table 2).

Table 2 – Modified Oxford Grading System for pelvic floor muscle strength [11]

Score	Finding
0	No contraction
1	Flicker
2	Weak
3	Moderate
4	Good
5	Strong

INVESTIGATIONS

Initial Tests

Perform urinalysis and MSU culture if appropriate.

If UTI present, treat with antibiotics and reassess urinary incontinence following successful treatment.

US urinary tract may be performed to assess PVR and hydronephrosis.

Consider flexible cystoscopy for persistent / severe symptoms, red-flag symptoms (visible haematuria and painful bladder), rUTI and voiding difficulties.

Pad Testing

The objective of a pad test is to try to quantify the volume of urine lost by weighing a perineal pad before and after provocation testing.

Pad test can be done as

- short term (1 hour), drink 500mL then proceed with exercise, ≤1.4g gain is normal
- or long term (24 hour), undergoing normal daily activity, ≤ 8g gain is normal

NICE do not recommend pad testing as routine assessment of women with urinary incontinence. [12]

Further Tests

UDS is the mainstay investigation for assessing severe / refractory OAB symptoms.

UDS need not be performed to investigate uncomplicated OAB / UI / SUI.

Lifestyle measures, bladder re-training / pelvic floor exercises and anticholinergics can be prescribed to treat presumed OAB without UDS.

NICE Guidelines suggest that UDS should be undertaken if: [12]
- symptoms of OAB leading to clinical suspicion of DO
- symptoms suggestive of voiding dysfunction
- previous surgery for SUI

Consider UDS prior to any surgical intervention (recall that 16% of SUI also have DO on UDS).

Consider VUDS if presenting with neurological features, in children or previous failed surgery.

MANAGEMENT

Prior to offering invasive treatment for either OAB or SUI, the patient should be discussed in the appropriate local urogynaecology / pelvic floor MDT.

MDT consists of sub-specialty interest urologist, urogynaecologist, physiotherapist, colorectal surgeon with special interest in functional bowel, continence nurse specialist. [12]

CONSERVATIVE MEASURES

The following behavioural measures should be considered: [12]
- optimisation of weight (weight loss improves UI in women)
- implementation of moderate exercise
- treatment of chronic cough / constipation
- smoking cessation (unlikely to benefit UI, advise as part of good medical practice)
- avoidance of caffeinated drinks (may improve urge symptoms but not UUI)

BLADDER RETRAINING

Bladder retraining is based on notion that central control can be re-learned as in infancy.

It is done by setting target time for using toilet before which patient should not void, gradually increasing intervals of time, whilst maintaining normal fluid intake.

Bladder retraining is effective for improvement of urinary incontinence in women.

Effectiveness diminishes after the treatment has ceased.

NICE (2019) recommend that bladder retraining be offered for ≥ 6 weeks as 1st line for UUI / MUI. [12]

PELVIC FLOOR MUSCLE TRAINING

The aim of PFMT is to strengthen and rehabilitate the pelvic floor, increase tone and urethral resistance however it may also inhibit bladder contraction in OAB (i.e. not only benefit incontinence).

Regime involves long slow contractions and short-sharp pull-ups at regular intervals.

NICE (2019) states PMFT should comprise ≥ 8 contractions performed 3x / day, for ≥ 3 months. [12]

PFMT may be undertaken electively in radical prostatectomy patients and pregnancy.

The addition of biofeedback to PFMT confers greater benefit in women.

PFMT is believed to benefit 30% of women with mild SUI.

Neurostimulation

NICE (2019) states that TENS should not be offered to treat OAB. [12]

ANTICHOLINERGICS

Anticholinergic drugs are mainstay of treatment for UUI and OAB.

The agents differ in their pharmacological / kinetic profiles, however there is limited evidence to suggest that one drug is superior to any other for QOL improvement. [13–14]

All anticholinergic drugs are superior to placebo in treating urinary incontinence, however absolute size of effect is small.

The efficacy varies between 50–75% (they increase voided volume and decrease detrusor pressure).

Higher doses are more effective but with a higher risk of side effects.

There is no demonstrable benefit in adding PFMT to anticholinergic drugs in treating UUI.

Adherence is low and most patients will stop treatment within first 3 months (due to lack of efficacy and / or side effects and / or cost).

Commonest side effect of anti-cholinergic drugs is dry mouth – others include constipation, blurred vision (accommodation paralysis), fatigue, cognitive dysfunction, prolonged QT interval.

Contra-indications to ACN use include:
- myasthenia gravis
- uncontrolled narrow-angle glaucoma
- bladder outflow obstruction / high risk of urinary retention
- active ulcerative colitis / toxic megacolon
- bowel obstruction or intestinal atony

Anticholinergics licensed for use in neurogenic bladders include trospium, oxybutynin and propiverine.

Mechanism of Action

Acetylcholine acts on muscarinic receptors on bladder smooth muscle causing contractions.

Majority of muscarinic receptors in the detrusor muscle are M2 (however M3 are the functionally important receptors).

Anticholinergic drugs are competitive muscarinic receptor antagonists and have high binding affinity mediating bladder contraction and reducing spontaneous detrusor activity during filling phase.

Selective anticholinergics block M1 / 2 receptors but not brain M1 receptors, thus are associated with a better side effect profile.

Table 3 – Examples of anticholinergic drugs and their properties [1]

Trade / Generic Name	Dosage	Receptor Selectivity	Half-life
Detrusitol / Tolterodine	2mg BD	Non-selective	2.4
Detrusitol XL / Tolterodine	4mg OD	Non-selective	8.4
Regurin / Trospium chloride	20mg BD	Non-selective	20
Ditropan / Oxybutynin chloride	2.5–5mg BD – QDS	Non-selective	2.3
Vesicare / Solifenacin	5–10mg OD	Selective M2 / M3	40–68

Anticholinergics and Dementia

It is believed that anticholinergic drugs have an association with cognitive dysfunction in the elderly.

This effect is not reversible, cumulative in nature and increases with length of exposure, and is therefore termed as "anti-cholinergic burden". [15]

Oxybutynin in particular has been shown to worsen cognition in adults.

Small molecular size and high lipophilicity are characteristics that increase ability of drug to cross the blood brain barrier.

US Study of ACN drugs and dementia (2015) described: [16]

- 3500 patients without dementia followed over 10-year period
- 1.5x increased risk of dementia for those taking ACN drugs regularly for 3 years
- relationship was dose-dependent and risk earned at any point of using medication

MIRABEGRON

Mirabegron is first clinically available β3-agonist drug.

β3-adrenoreceptors are the predominant β-receptors in detrusor smooth muscle cells and their stimulation is thought to induce detrusor relaxation.

Mirabegron is better than placebo and has similar efficacy to anticholinergic drugs. [17]

Adverse events with mirabegron are similar to placebo.

Contra-indications to mirabegron use include:
- severe uncontrolled hypertension (systolic BP ≥ 180mmHg, diastolic BP ≥ 110mmHg)
- known hypersensitivity to agent

Avoid usage in severe liver impairment and renal impairment (eGFR < 30mL / min / 1.73m^2).

Standard dose is 50mg OD (reduce to 25mg in mild liver impairment).

Side-effects of mirabegron use include:
- arrhythmias
- UTI / cystitis
- dyspepsia, skin reactions, joint swelling
- hypertensive crisis (rare)

If pharmacological therapy (anticholinergics and / or mirabegron) fails, the next step in the management of OAB is referral for UDS.

VAGINAL OESTROGEN TREATMENT

Topical local vaginal oestrogen treatment is primarily used to treat OAB symptoms due to vaginal atrophy in post-menopausal women. [12]

It is not associated with the increased risks of VTE and breast cancer that is seen in systemic oestrogen administration.

It improves urinary incontinence for post-menopausal women in the short-term and should be offered.

Vaginal oestrogen should be prescribed on long-term basis – breast cancer is not an absolute contra-indication however if history is positive the attending oncologist should be consulted first.

Ideal length of treatment remains unclear.

An example of a suitable vaginal oestrogen treatment regime includes:
- consider first choice Estriol 0.01% cream
- apply once daily for 2–3 weeks,
- then reduced to twice weekly,
- discontinue every 2–3 months for 4 weeks to reassess need for further treatment

BOTULINUM TOXIN

Botulinum toxin is a neurotoxin derived from clostridium botulinum.

There are 7 serotypes all with similar pharmacological effects – types A and B are for clinical use (BOTOX is botulinum toxin A and 5x more potent than Dysport®).

BOTOX is indicated for treating:

- NDO / IDO / DetSD
- where these conditions have previously been proven by VUDS and are refractory to conservative / medical therapy

The mean efficacy for treating IDO is 70%, and effect seen for 4–10 months (mean 6 months).

Botulinum A is much more effective in treating NDO compared to IDO.

Side-effects include:

- urinary retention (10% risk in IDO, higher in NDO 30–40%)
- UTI, bladder pain, haematuria

Contra-indications to BoNT/A use include:

- myasthenia gravis
- concurrent use of amino-glycosides (e.g. gentamicin) which may augment effects
- Eaton-Lambert syndrome (autoimmune condition causing limb muscle weakness due to antibodies against pre-synaptic calcium channels at neuromuscular junction)
- breast-feeding / pregnancy
- bleeding disorders
- inability to perform ISC

Tolerance to the drug appears unchanged with repeated applications.

DIGNITY Study [18]

Randomised, double-blind placebo-controlled multi-centre study designed to evaluate the effects of onabotulinumtoxinA on urinary incontinence, UDS and QOL in NDO.

MS (n = 154) and SCI (n = 121) randomised to placebo vs. 200units vs. 300units (1:1:1)

Primary end-point – change from baseline in urinary incontinence episodes after 6 weeks

Secondary end-point – QOL score, UDS maximum cystometric capacity

Findings – significant reduction in urinary incontinence episodes and improved QOL in treatment groups, however no significant difference noted between doses

EMBARK Study [19]

Randomised placebo-controlled trial studying OAB patients who failed anticholinergic treatment

> 500 patients who had ≥ 3 urinary incontinence episodes in 3 days were randomised to placebo vs. 100units onabotulinumtoxinA.

Primary outcome was change in incontinence episodes, secondary end-point was QOL.

Findings – treatment group superior in all OAB symptoms and QOL end-points

Mechanism of Action

Botulinum toxin A temporarily blocks pre-synaptic release of acetylcholine at the neuromuscular junction of the parasympathetic nerves supplying the detrusor resulting in temporary paralysis.

It also prevents the exocytosis of acetylcholine by cleaving SNAP-25 off the SNARE proteins (a complex protein which when intact forms the core of neuro-exocytosis machinery).

The resulting chemical denervation is a reversible process.

Administration

BOTOX given intra-detrusor via flexible / rigid cystoscope with local / general anaesthesia

The standard starting dose for IDO is 100units, for NDO it is higher at 200units.

Avoid trigonal area for injection and intra-detrusor rather than submucosal technique is preferred, no consensus regarding number of injection sites.

Do not give with gentamicin (aminoglycosides) as can potentiate action of BOTOX and cause systemic effects (consider cefuroxime).

NICE (2019) Guidance [12]

BOTOX should be authorised by pelvic floor MDT for OAB caused by DO on UDS where pharmacological therapy has failed, and the patient should be able to perform ISC.

Offer 100units of botulinum toxin A as starting dose for OAB in women – if symptom relief is inadequate, consider increasing dose to 200units.

Do not offer botulinum toxin type B to women with OAB.

POSTERIOR TIBIAL NERVE STIMULATION

The PTNS device is connected near the ankle to stimulate the posterior tibial nerve, such that impulses travel to the sacral nerve plexus to modulate bladder function.

NICE (2019) recommends that PTNS can be offered provided: [12]

- This has been authorised by the local relevant MDT
- Non-surgical / pharmacological management has not been successful
- Female patient does not want botulinum toxin A or SNM

There is no current guidance on the use of PTNS in men.

SACRAL NEUROMODULATION

NICE (2019) advises SNM can be offered to patients: [12]

- with OAB refractory to non-surgical management including medicines
- provided this has been authorised by local MDT
- botulinum toxin A unsuccessful or patient unwilling to accept the potential risk of ISC

SNM is also known as sacral nerve stimulation.

SNM works by continuous mild electrical stimulation of afferents to bladder (mainly S3) modulating local neural reflexes and inhibits bladder contraction.

SNM also affects higher brain centres involved in control of micturition.

Success rates ≤ 70%

The side-effects of SNM insertion include:

- local complications of bleeding and infection
- pain at the site of implantation

- discomfort in ankle or foot
- adverse effect on bowel function
- device infection requiring removal

SNM Insertion

Can be performed under general or local anaesthesia

A two-stage technique is recommended to improve efficacy from 50% to 75%.
- initially a test stimulation wire is inserted into S3 foramina attached to temporary external pulse generator device
- patient is discharged and asked to keep a bladder diary for ≥ 2 weeks
- if improvement of ≥ 50% is noted, proceed to insert a permanent electrode is into S3 foramen with pulse generator in pouch superficial to posterior superior iliac crest

Bilateral S3 nerve root stimulation for SNM has been proposed as an alternative for failed unilateral lead placement, however the efficacy of this remains to be proven.

If patient experiences post-operative pain after insertion, consider:
- signs of infection?
- switch off SNM device (if pain settles this suggest it is due to electrical output)
- if no change by turning off, suggests cause is "pocket related" (e.g. size, erosion, seroma)

If symptoms return after an initial period of efficacy, check the battery and assess for lead migration by means of on XR.

A patient will not be able to have an MRI scan after they have an SNM inserted.

CLAM AUGMENTATION CYSTOPLASTY

In clam augmentation cystoplasty the bladder is bi-valved (i.e. opened coronally) and the defect is patched with a segment of bowel.

The most common segment used is the distal ileum (usually 25cm segment, starting 25cm proximal to the ileocaecal valve.

Any bowel segment can in theory be used if it has appropriate mesenteric length.

Cystoplasty will impair bladder contraction, lower detrusor pressures and increase bladder capacity.

The contra-indications for performing CAC include: [1]
- severe inflammatory bowel disease
- previous pelvic radiotherapy
- short bowel
- inability to perform CISC
- significant renal impairment (cannot compensate hyperchloraemic metabolic acidosis)
- significant hepatic impairment

The post-operative complications of CAC include: [1]
- pain / infection / bleeding
- wound dehiscence / fistula
- MI / VTE / anaesthetic complications
- small bowel obstruction / anastomotic leak
- mortality ≤ 2.5%

Long-term CAC Sequalae

Need for CISC – increases over time

Stones – more common in context of Mitrofanoff

Mucus production – remains constant over time and can lead to rUTI, stones, blockages

Bacteriuria – almost 100% of patients will have asymptomatic bacteriuria

Deterioration of renal function

Bladder perforation – high associated mortality due to frequent delay in diagnosis

Increase risk of cancer – a longer term risk, usually adenocarcinoma in the region of the anastomosis

Bowel changes – diarrhoea and low B12 / folate (no terminal ileum absorption)

Reduced growth potential – the H⁺ (from the acidosis) is buffered in exchange for Ca^{2+} causing bone demineralisation (osteopaenia)

CAC Biochemical Sequalae

Ammonium chloride (NH_4Cl) is absorbed by the clammed bowel segment ➜ NH_3 + HCl

HCl ➜ H+ + Cl- (i.e. hyperchloraemic acidosis)

The acidosis is usually not clinically important (however if significant then treat with bicarbonate).

This similar problem does not happen in context of ileal conduit, because the urine passes through and therefore does not have the time to be absorbed (cystoplasty is a reservoir).

STRESS INCONTINENCE

SUI is the involuntary leakage of urine on effort / exertion.

50% of all urinary incontinence in women is SUI; this is bothersome to 20% of those with it.

Urodynamic stress incontinence is noted during UDS and defined as involuntary leakage of urine during increases in abdominal pressure in absence of detrusor contraction.

Intrinsic sphincter deficiency is the primary underlying cause for SUI in women (extrinsic urethral sphincter is not the primary mechanism for continence).

DIAGNOSTIC EVALUATION

PATIENT HISTORY

The patient should be seen in dedicated functional urology clinic with continence nurse specialist.

Consider prior completion of bladder diary over ≥ 3 days, a validated symptom questionnaire e.g. ICIQ-SF (see "Overactive Bladder" station), urinalysis, PVR assessment.

A thorough history should be taken, as above, regarding SUI in particular:
- distinguish between SUI, UUI or MUI
- identify SUI risk factors (obesity, chronic cough / constipation, multiple vaginal deliveries with instrumentation, previous pelvic surgery / radiotherapy, oestrogen withdrawal
- assess for neurological conditions
- past urological history

PATIENT EXAMINATION

All patient examinations should be performed in the presence of a chaperone.

Examination should be performed as per "Overactive Bladder", however regarding SUI in particular:
- abdomen, for palpable bladder, scars

- supine pelvic, for oestrogen status, cough test, pelvic floor tone assessment
- left lateral position, for cystocoele and rectocele
- peripheral neurology and lower spine

INVESTIGATIONS

Initial Tests

Perform urinalysis and MSU culture if appropriate.

If UTI present, treat with antibiotics and reassess the UI following successful treatment.

US urinary tract may be performed to assess for PVR and hydronephrosis.

Consider flexible cystoscopy for persistent / severe symptoms, red-flag symptoms (visible haematuria and painful bladder), rUTI and voiding difficulties.

NICE (2019) do not recommend pad testing as part of routine assessment for women with UI. [12]

NICE (2019) do not recommend that UDS must be performed to investigate uncomplicated SUI. [12]

Lifestyle measures, bladder re-training / pelvic floor exercises can be prescribed to treat presumed SUI without prior UDS.

NICE Guidelines suggest that UDS should be undertaken to investigate SUI if: [12]

- symptoms leading to clinical suspicion of concomitant DO
- symptoms suggestive of voiding dysfunction
- previous surgery for SUI

Consider UDS prior to any SUI surgical intervention (recall that 16% of SUI also have DO on UDS)

- if VLPP < 60cm H_2O, consider intrinsic sphincter deficiency
- if VLPP > 90cm H_2O, consider anatomical cause

The Blaivas and Olson classification was a tool developed to classify SUI based on VUDS / fluoroscopic imaging, describing the position of the bladder neck and urethra, and is occasionally used. [20]

MANAGEMENT

Prior to offering invasive treatment for either OAB or SUI, the patient should be discussed in the appropriate local urogynaecology MDT.

Patient should be provided with BAUS leaflet or NICE Patient decision aid describing all options of incontinence treatment.

Surgical options include: bulking agents vs. autologous sling vs. colposuspension vs. AUS.

CONSERVATIVE MEASURES

Lifestyle advice is paramount and should be discussed:
- weight loss, exercise, dietary advice
- smoking cessation / treatment of chronic cough and constipation
- fluid intake – avoid caffeinated drinks, moderate volumes

Further non-surgical strategies as discussed previously include:
- supervised pelvic floor exercises
- bladder re-training
- topical local oestrogen therapy (if evidence of vaginal atrophy)

The patient should be referred to the community continence team for implementation and supervision of the advice above.

DULOXETINE

Duloxetine is the only agent with published data available as medical therapy for SUI.

Duloxetine inhibits pre-synaptic re-uptake of neurotransmitters (serotonin 5-HT and norepinephrine) at the spinal cord level (Onuf's nucleus). [21]

Mechanism of action is to increase activity of pudendal nerve and urethral muscle tone.

Prescribed as 20–40mg BD (PO)

Side-effects are common and limit use:
- dry mouth, constipation, nausea
- dizziness, insomnia and fatigue

Duloxerine is not advised as 1st line treatment for SUI due to side-effect profile, rather as 2nd line or alternative option to surgery if patient is unfit or unwilling.

BULKING AGENTS

The injection of bulking materials into bladder neck and peri-urethral muscles is a minimally invasive technique to increase outlet resistance.

Main indication is SUI in women due to intrinsic sphincter deficiency with normal detrusor function.

Other indications include patient preference, medically unfit for surgery, previous failed procedures and mild / moderate SUI.

Contra-indicated if active UTI, concomitant DO and bladder neck stenosis

The *complications* of injection of bulking agents includes:
- temporary urinary retention requiring ISC (10%)
- failure to improve symptoms / need for further injections (≤ 50%)
- UTI / haematuria

Results tend to deteriorate with time and repeat treatments often needed.

Bulking agents are less effective than surgery for treating SUI (however lower complication rates) and should not be offered to those patients seeking permanent cure.

No bulking agent is known to be superior to any other, consider macroplastique (silicone) as there is no significant risk of migration due to particle size.

Procedure

The procedure for injecting bulking agent in FRCS (Urol) viva:
- WHO checklist complete and patient prepped, draped in supine lithotomy position
- Induction IV gentamicin antibiotic
- Perform full diagnostic cystoscopy
- 2mg bulkamid given in 4 divided doses (at 12′, 3′, 6′ and 9′ o'clock) 1cm distal to bladder neck

NICE (2019) advise efficacy is inferior to synthetic tapes / autologous slings. [12]

MID-URETHRAL SLINGS

Mid-urethral slings are most frequently used surgical intervention for SUI in Europe.

They work by impeding the movement of the posterior urethral wall.

MUS can be classified into:
- *autologous*: rectus fascia, fascia lata
- *synthetic*: proline, Dacron
- *allograft* / cadaveric

Synthetic slings can be placed via retro-pubic (TVT) or trans-obturator (TOT) routes as day case.

Concerns regarding Vaginal Mesh

The initial MHRA review concluded that synthetic mesh insertion is permissible provided:
- the patient must be warned of potential complications
- process is audited on recognised database (e.g. BAUS)
- adverse event report should be sent to MHRA
- any mesh removal should be undertaken in a centre with specialist expertise

However there have since been concerns raised regarding use of synthetic mesh in vaginal implants for prolapse and SUI surgery, which has led to a pause in their use.

Trans-Vaginal Tape (TVT)

The TVT procedure is carried out as follows:
- WHO checklist complete and patient prepped, draped in supine lithotomy position
- Induction IV gentamicin antibiotic
- full diagnostic rigid cystoscopy to identify both UOs (insert catheter)
- small midline anterior vaginal incision over mid-urethra
- insert trocar either side of urethra, perforate endo-pelvic fascia, push out above pubis

- position tape loosely (tension free) over mid-urethra
- remove outer tape coverings, cut flush to skin, check cystoscopy for bladder injury

The *complications* of TVT slings include:
- bladder perforation (≤ 10%)
- severe bleeding (1%)
- injury to blood vessels / bowel / nerve
- material related e.g. erosion / migration into urethra, bladder, rectum (1%)
- voiding dysfunction including urinary retention (5%) permanent / temporary, ongoing SUI

Efficacy of TVT is 90% (1 year) and ≤ 80% (5 years).

Trans-Obturator Tape

TOT surgery performed initially as per TVT, however outer incisions are lateral to labia major at level of clitoris and tape passes through obturator foramen.

TVT vs. TOT have equivalent patient-reported outcomes (cure rates).

Compared to TVT, the TOT procedure has:
- lower risk of bladder perforation and voiding dysfunction
- higher risk of vaginal injuries, groin / thigh pain and mesh erosion

Tape Erosion

Tape must be removed if there is a urethral or vaginal erosion.

Martius fat pad can be used to close urethral defects if significant.

Bladder migration / perforation can be attempted to be removed cystoscopically, or with laser, if considerable defect then may need open cystostomy.

Autologous Slings

Most commonly a segment of rectus fascia measuring 10–20cm in length is harvested via Pfannensteil incision, non-absorbable long sutures placed on both ends.

The sling is placed under mid-urethra.

Sutures placed through endopelvic fascia up to remaining rectus tied using correct tension.

Autologous slings are more effective than colposuspension for improving SUI, at the expense of higher rates of complication (voiding dysfunction).

Colposuspension

Retropubic suspension surgery used to treat female SUI mainly caused by urethral hyper-mobility.

The surgical principle is re-elevation of bladder neck into the abdominal pressure zone so there is equal transmission of pressure to bladder neck to close off the urethra.

The following patients may benefit from colposuspension:

- young patient with SUI (due to current concerns regarding long-term use of mesh)
- SUI with significant urethral hyper-mobility

Burch colposuspension is the most widely used procedure for this purpose.

Burch colposuspension has longest follow up (69% cured for > 10 years). [22]

It can be performed open or laparoscopically, with similar efficacy rates however open option has a longer in-patient stay and higher complication rate.

The procedure involves exposing para-vaginal fascia and approximating it to the Cooper's ligament of superior pubic rami.

The complications after Burch colposuspension include:

- immediate – retropubic space haemorrhage, bladder trauma
- *delayed* – rectocoele ($\leq$ 20%), dyspareunia, voiding dysfunction / CISC, rUTI

The alternative Marshall-Marchetti-Krantz procedure is not recommended by NICE.

Penile Clamps

Urethral compression devices used in men with pure sphincteric incompetence (e.g. post-RP)

Rarely used due to modern alternatives such as the AUS; an option if the patient is medically unfit.

Applied at the lowest pressure to relieve incontinence, must be unclamped every 3–4 hours and not to be worn at night.

POST-PROSTATECTOMY INCONTINENCE

DIAGNOSTIC EVALUATION

PATIENT HISTORY

The history for evaluating sphincter damage and symptoms should include:
- causative procedure – RP, TURP, pelvic radiotherapy, pelvic fracture
- details of cancer status e.g. PSA, margin status, planned adjuvant treatments
- symptomatology, distinguishing SUI from UUI and impact on QOL
- erectile function
- overall fitness, hand function and cognitive status

Patient should be encouraged to complete ICIQ-SF questionnaire (or equivalent) prior to clinic.

Patient should complete bladder diary.

Duration of symptoms following RP is important, most patients will have regained their continence within 12 months of surgery.

PATIENT EXAMINATION

Perform urinalysis (and MSU as appropriate) – if positive, treat and reassess.

To confirm the diagnosis after RP for example, perform:
- abdominal examination, for palpable bladder
- cough test

Further imaging may include US for assessment of PVR.

The key investigation is VUDS, which typically reveals stable compliant bladder with evidence of SUI.

If a pad test is performed over 24 hours, leakage of < 200mL / day (mild), 200–500mL / day (moderate) and > 500mL / day (severe).

MANAGEMENT

All conservative options should be advised initially:

- weight loss, exercise, diet, smoking cessation
- supervised PFMT
- bladder retraining
- consider duloxetine with counselling regarding side effects

After failure of conservative methods and sufficient time for natural continence recovery, men with post-prostatectomy incontinence should be counselled regarding their options.

Bulking agents are only to be considered as a short-term option for temporary relief and should not be offered for severe PPI.

MALE SLINGS

Fixed slings have been introduced to treat post-prostatectomy incontinence.

These are positioned under the urethra and fixed by trans-obturator or retro-pubic approach, the tension adjusted during surgery which cannot be subsequently readjusted.

No particular sling has demonstrated superiority over others

ARTIFICIAL URETHRAL SPHINCTER

The AUS can be used for all degrees of post-prostatectomy incontinence.

The AUS is a closed pressurised system with 3 components:
- urethral cuff, placed around bulbar urethra or bladder neck
- activating control pump, placed in scrotum (or labia majora)
- reservoir, placed extra-peritoneally in the abdomen (provides constant pressure to cuff)

The cuff provides a constant circumferential pressure to compress the urethra and is derived from the reservoir which is normally set at 61–70cm H_2O.

To void, the pump is squeezed which transfers fluid to reservoir balloon, deflating the cuff which then refills within 3 minutes (the time interval during which patient must void).

Efficacy is 75% completely dry and 90% socially continent, 60% have benefits for > 10 years.

The complications of AUS insertion include:

- infection (most common pathogen is Staph. epidermidis)
- cuff erosion, urethral atrophy (most common cause of surgical revision)
- persistent leakage, mechanical failure

Atrophy presents with gradual de-novo onset of incontinence, mechanical failure tends to present with sudden onset incontinence.

Erosions / infections of AUS require removal, do not reinsert for ≥ 3 months.

Always ensure the AUS is deactivated prior to any urethral instrumentation.

MASTER Trial

Male synthetic sling vs. AUS Trial is an RCT comparing the two post-prostatectomy treatment modalities in terms of effectiveness as well as cost and relative harms.

The trial aims to determine non-inferiority of the male sling when compared to AUS.

URODYNAMICS

UDS is the only method that can objectively assess LUT function.

In neuro-urological patients UDS interpretation can be more challenging, and same session repeat UDS are crucial as repeat measurements may yield different results.

In patients with AD monitor the blood pressure during UDS.

DEFINITIONS

The following are useful definitions when interpreting UDS:

Bladder compliance, relationship between change in bladder volume (ΔV) and change in detrusor pressure (ΔP_{det}), where compliance is ($\Delta V / \Delta P_{det}$)

Cystometric capacity (bladder volume), urine volume at the end of the filling phase

Detrusor overactivity, involuntary detrusor contractions during filling phase (diagnosis of DO can be made irrespective of the size of the contractions)

Neurogenic DO, is DO in presence of underlying neurological condition

Terminal DO, single detrusor contraction at cystometric capacity which results in flooding

Detrusor sphincter dyssynergia, detrusor contraction concurrent with involuntary contraction of urethral striated muscle which affects flow

Abdominal leak point pressure, intra-vesical pressure at which urine leakage occurs due to increased abdominal pressure in absence of detrusor contraction

Detrusor leak point pressure, the lower detrusor pressure at which urine leakage occurs

Urethral pressure, the fluid pressure needed to just open a closed urethra

Urethra pressure profile, a graph indicating intraluminal pressure along length of urethra

INDICATIONS

There are many indications for performing UDS, including:
- persistent LUTS after appropriate therapy (e.g. BOO surgery)
- previous failed incontinence surgery

- mixed urinary symptoms +/- incontinence
- suspicion of underlying neurological disease and urinary symptoms
- children with complex voiding dysfunction

VUDS should be used in neuro-urological patients.

In patients with new SCI, once the upper tracts are safe (e.g. SPC, LTC) they should be referred for UDS to provide baseline trace as they are at risk of neuropathic bladder changes in the future.

Contraindications to performing UDS include:
- active use of pharmacotherapy for bladder dysfunction (pause 48 hours before)
- active UTI (study should be postponed)
- perform with caution in AD

TECHNIQUE

UDS should be performed in dedicated room with specialised equipment (VUDS requires fluoroscopy).

Perform urinalysis to exclude infection prior to commencing the study.

1. Uroflowmetry and PVR

Begin with flow rate test to provide a first impression of voiding function. [1]

2. UDS Setup

Clean external urethral meatus, pass anaesthetic gel, insert dual-lumen 6–8F catheter into the bladder (to record intra-vesical pressure) and drain bladder (note the PVR).

Insert single-lumen catheter into rectum to record abdominal pressure.

Connect lines to urodynamic transducers and flush these with saline to remove any air bubbles.

Zero all lines to atmosphere, place transducers at level of pubic symphysis. Make patient cough several times to ensure adequate subtraction (P_{det} < 6cm / H_2O at rest at the start).

Detrusor pressure (P_{det}) = (intra-vesical pressure) − (abdominal pressure)

3. Filling Cystometry

Only means for quantifying the patient's filling function – start with empty bladder.

Fill slowly at physiological rate 20mL/min for neuropaths, 50mL/min for adults) using warm saline (or contrast medium in VUDS), cough every minute to review subtraction.

Normal pressures at rest: P_{det} 0–6cm H_2O, Pves and Pabd 15–40cm H_2O

Note the following findings on the filling phase:

- volume of first sensation, first urge and strong desire, cystometric capacity
- evidence of involuntary detrusor contractions (DO)
- evidence of slow rising intra-vesical pressure (poor compliance)
- incontinence and precipitating cause (SUI or UUI)

Filling phase historically described as having 4 distinct parts: [image 2]

I. initial fill (unfolding, viscoelastic)
II. tonus phase (viscoelastic)
III. limit of compliance (viscoelastic properties exhausted)
IV. voiding (now considered to be in voiding phase)

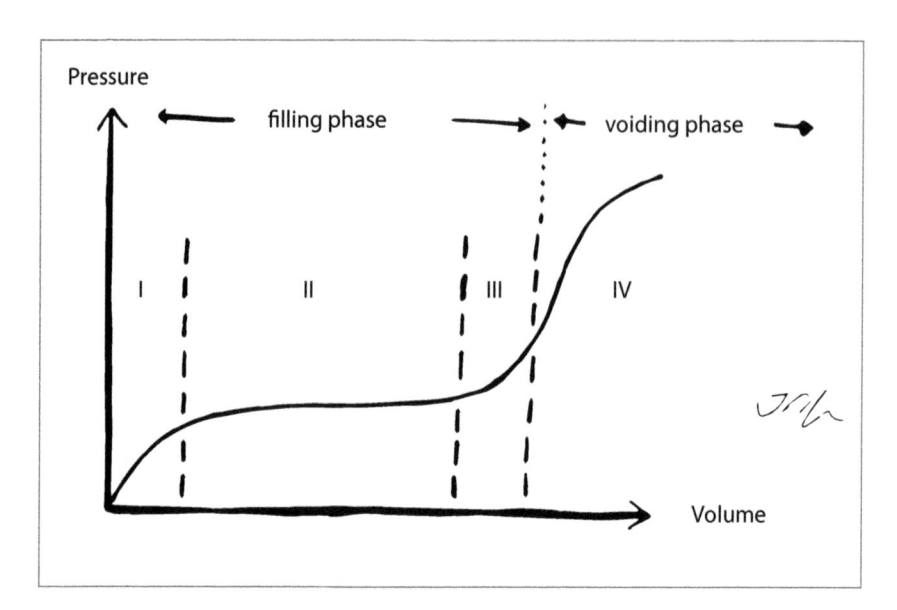

Image 2 – Distinct parts of the filling phase on UDS

4. Voiding Cystometry

Pressure flow studies during the voiding phase reflects the co-ordination between detrusor and urethra / pelvic floor – VUDS and filling phase should be interpreted alongside this.

Note the following findings on the voiding phase:
- P_{det} at Q_{max} and Q_{max} (determine BOO, bladder contractility index, detrusor failure)
- voiding time and shape of curve
- reciprocal relationship between voiding curve and P_{det} (DetSD)

Bladder contractility index = $P_{det}Q_{max} + 5Q_{max}$

    BCI >150 = strong contractility

    BCI 100–150 = normal contractility

    BCI <100 = weak contractility

Bladder contractility nomogram – the patient can be plotted on the nomogram to determine whether their BCI is weak, normal or strong. [Figure 1] [23]

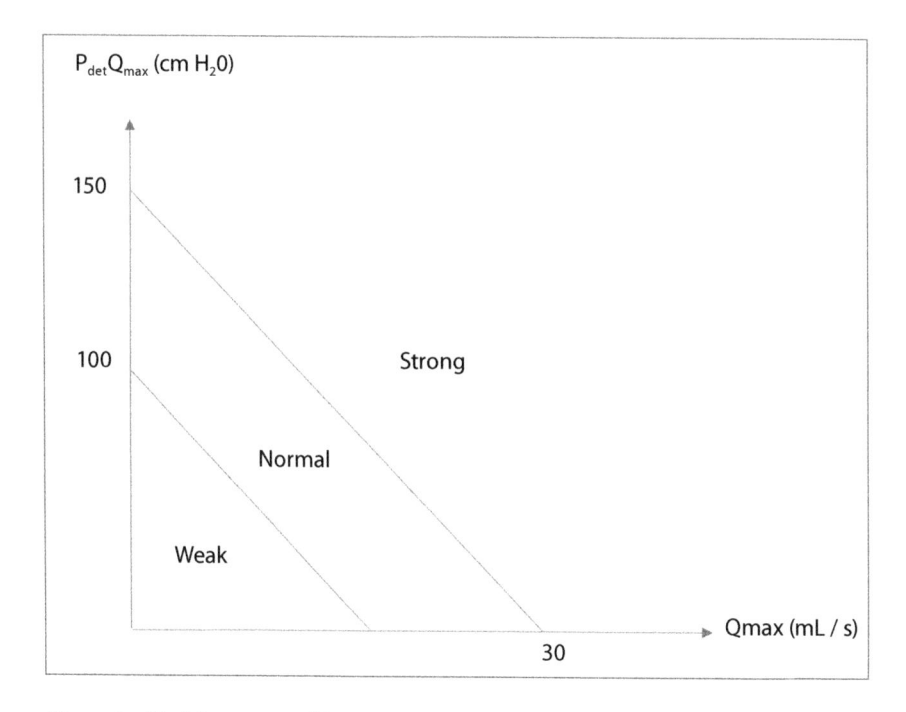

Figure 1 – Bladder contractility nomogram

Bladder outlet obstruction index (also Abrams-Griffiths number) = $(P_{det}Q_{max}) - (2Q_{max})$

BOOI >40 = obstructed

BOOI 20–40 = equivocal

BOOI <20 = non-obstructed

The ICS nomogram can be used to plot the measurements during UDS to determine whether the patient is obstructed, unobstructed or in the equivocal range.

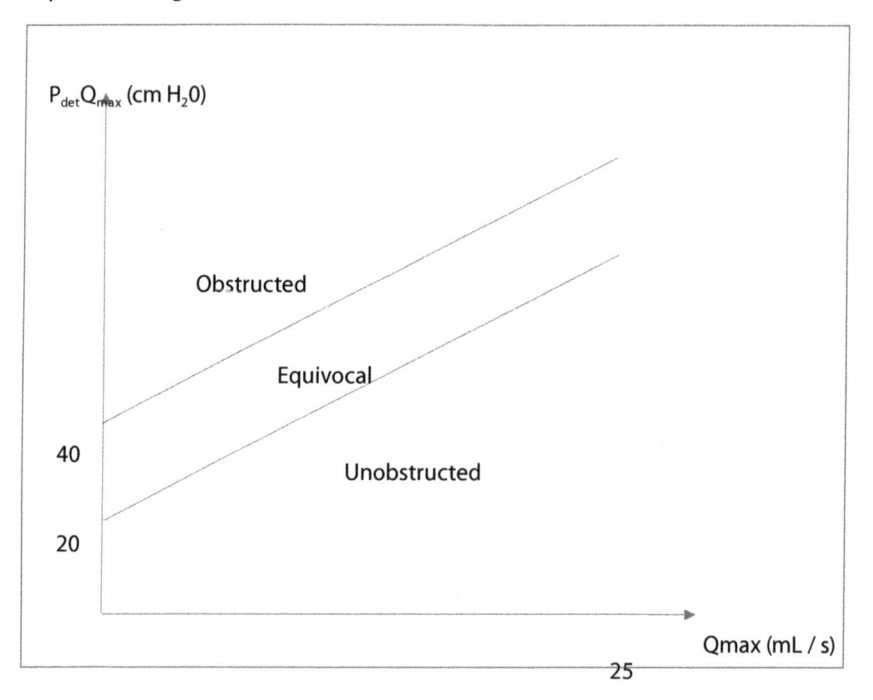

Figure 2 – Bladder outflow obstruction nomogram

Loss of compliance is defined as > 1cm H_2O rise in pressure per 40mL infused, standardised ≤ 400mL (i.e. no more than 10cm H_2O rise in pressure should be noted during filling).

The definitions and nomograms that are used to describe BOO in men do not apply to women.

In women there is no condition as common as BPH and therefore developing nomograms by similar methods is difficult. [24]

Causes of obstruction in women vary from anatomical (e.g. POP) to functional (e.g. dysfunctional voiding) without one predominant diagnosis.

5. Leak Point Pressures

DLPP is the lowest detrusor pressure at which urine leakage occurs in the absence of either a detrusor contraction or increased abdominal pressure.

This term applies and should only be used in relation to neuropathic patients.

DLPP gives an indication of fixed outlet resistance.

DLPP > 40cm H_2O is associated with increased risk of upper tract dilatation and deterioration.

ALPP (also Valsalva leak point pressure), intravesical pressure at which leakage occurs because of increased abdominal pressure in absence of detrusor contraction.

ALPP is important in the investigation of SUI:

    ALPP < 60 cm H_2O = significant intrinsic sphincter deficiency

    ALPP > 90 cm H_2O = SUI likely due to urethral hypermobility

    ALPP > 150 cm H_2O = urethra unlikely to be the cause of UI

DETRUSOR SPHINCTER DYSSYNERGIA

DetSD is the involuntary contraction of the urethral and / or peri-urethral striated muscle simultaneously with detrusor contractions.

DetSD is usually specific to supra sacral neurological injuries or disorders.

Classic UDS trace in DetSD is "saw-tooth appearance" on P_{det} line and sustained (e.g. >5 minutes) detrusor contractions with pressures 80–90 cm H_2O).

Cystography at VUDS reveal a hold-up of contrast at the level of the external urethral sphincter.

DSD is dangerous for the upper tracts due to the high-pressure system.

The treatment aim is to reduce the pressures within the bladder to safeguard the upper tracts and avoid development of nephropathy.

Management

Aim is to achieve low-pressure storage, complete bladder emptying and promote continence.

Commence anticholinergic medication, teach patient CISC (or pass LTC)

and monitor closely with repeat US at 3 months looking for upper tract dilatation.

Repeat UDS after 3–6 months to ensure bladder pressures have come down.

Intra-detrusor BOTOX is an option; however the patient would still need to perform CISC.

Augmentation cystoplasty +/- Mitrofanoff channel is an option, however the patient would still need to perform CISC.

VUDS should be repeated 3–6 months after cystoplasty.

Urethral stents (placed across the external urethral sphincter) or external sphincterotomy can treat DetSD, however the patient will suffer with continuous incontinence thereafter.

Sacral anterior nerve root stimulator abolished the reflex bladder, increases capacity, abolishes AD but leads to SUI and loss of reflex erections.

FEMALE URETHRAL DIVERTICULUM

A FUD is an epithelialized outpouching of the urethral mucosa with a single connection (ostium) entering the urethral lumen. [25]

Multiple in 10% of cases

Most common malignancy found in a FUD is adenocarcinoma.

AETIOLOGY

Believed to arise secondary to infection of peri-urethral glands, leading to local abscess formation and eventual rupture into the lumen

Glands are located posterolateral to peri-urethral fascia (proximal 2 / 3) and drain into distal 1 / 3.

FUD is rarely congenital, however common acquired causes include:
- traumatic vaginal delivery
- previous urethral / vaginal surgery
- repeated urethral instrumentation
- peri-urethral (Skene's) gland infection (e.g. N.gonorrhoea, E.coli)

FUD can be single, saddle-shaped or even circumferential.

DIAGNOSTIC EVALUATION

PATIENT HISTORY

FUD presents with classic "three D's" (dyspareunia, dribble post-void, dysuria) only in 23% of cases.

In clinical practice patients present with a wide range of symptoms, enquire regarding:
- dysuria, dribble post-void, dyspareunia
- rUTI, visible haematuria, urgency
- previous STI / instrumentation / local abscesses / previous urethro-vaginal surgery

PATIENT EXAMINATION

Pelvic examination is essential – always ensure presence of female chaperone.

Look for anterior midline vaginal wall mass which may be palpable and may discharge fluid (culture this as appropriate).

Perform urinalysis.

IMAGING

MRI is the gold-standard diagnostic imaging for diagnosing FUD. [1]

Sensitivity approaches 100% when used with endo-vaginal coil (i.e. not a surface coil technique) and allows localisation for surgical planning.

US (trans- vaginal / rectal / perineal) accuracy is operator dependent.

MCUG has good sensitivity and allows concomitant assessment of any voiding dysfunction, however the test exposes patient to radiation.

CYSTOSCOPY

Use 0° or 30° scope and perform full diagnostic cystoscopy to check for other pathology.

Compress anterior vaginal wall with finger in vagina and inspect urethral lumen for any expressed pus from the urethra.

MANAGEMENT

Asymptomatic FUD does not require active intervention.

Patients should be adequately counselled regarding clinical course of condition and symptoms to monitor and need not be followed up.

Patients with LUTS, rUTI or pain symptoms may benefit from FUD surgery.

The principles of FUD repair include:
- excision of diverticulum
- closure of connection to the ostium
- water-tight urethral closure +/- inter-positioned Martius fat pad
- preservation of continence (or alternatively insertion of sling device)
- catheterisation for ≤ 14 days

Complications from FUD repair include incontinence, urethra-vaginal fistula, urethral stricture, recurrent diverticulae and scarring leading to dyspareunia.

FEMALE URINARY TRACT FISTULAE

VESICOVAGINAL FISTULAE

The most common type of urinary tract fistula is VVF.

The most common cause of VVF in developing countries is obstructed labour, due to ischaemic necrosis of the anterior vaginal wall. [26]

VVF can be evaluated using dye method – oral pyridium (turns urine orange) +/- intra-vesical methylene blue as double dye test (evaluate colour present on inserted vaginal tampon).

Surgical Management

Options for repair of VVF are abdominal vs. vaginal.

Success rates between the two techniques are comparable. [27]

Abdominal repair associated with greater length of in-patient stay and morbidity; however it preserves vaginal depth.

Vaginal repair has a lower associated morbidity and risk of ureteric injury, however a greater risk of vaginal shortening.

A Martius labial fat flap should be used (blood supply from external pudendal artery).

COLOVESICAL FISTULAE

The most common cause of colovesical fistulae is diverticular disease (colon cancer second most).

CT imaging should reveal air in the bladder, diverticulosis, with an area of thickened bladder next to a loop of thickened bowel (confirm findings with cystoscopy).

VESICOUTERINE FISTULAE

Vesicoutrerine fistulae occur most commonly after "Lower Segment Caesarean" station.

If fertility is not important to the patient, proceed to hysterectomy. Fertility preserving options include observation, cystoscopy and fulguration of fistula tract, repair with interposition of omental flap.

PELVIC ORGAN PROLAPSE

AETIOLOGY

The congenital causes of POP include:
- connective tissue disorders e.g. Ehler-Dahlos syndrome,
- spina bifida

The acquired causes of POP include:
- previous vaginal surgery (prolapse repair, colposuspension, hysterectomy
- obesity, chronic cough / constipation
- previous vaginal delivery
- low oestrogen levels

Anterior wall prolapse, is herniation of bladder (cystocoele) or urethra (urethrocoele).

Posterior wall prolapse, is protrusion of rectum (rectocoele) or peritoneum (enterocoele).

Middle compartment prolapse, includes uterine prolapse or procidentia (entire uterus).

CLASSIFICATION

POP quantification (POPQ) is a validated system which allows standardisation of descriptions of POP by measuring distances between defined anatomical points and the hymen.

The ICS has a staging of POP which is based on the POPQ. [Table 4]

The Baden and Walker system provides a practical alternative classification tool. [Table 5]

Table 4 – ICS staging of pelvic organ prolapse [28]

Stage	Leading Edge of POP in relation to hymen	Description
0	< -3cm	No POP
1	< -1cm	POP > 1cm above hymen
2	≤ -1cm and ≥ 1cm	POP between 1cm above and below hymen
3	> 1cm and < 2cm	POP > 1cm below hymen, no vaginal eversion
4		Complete vaginal eversion

Table 5 – Baden and Walker classification of pelvic organ prolapse [28]

Grade	Description
0	No prolapse
1	Descent halfway to the hymen
2	Descent to hymen
3	Descent halfway past the hymen
4	Maximal descent / eversion

DIAGNOSTIC EVALUATION

PATIENT HISTORY

The history should enquire regarding symptoms of:
- vaginal pressure / bulge / heaviness or need for manual reduction
- positional variation (i.e. worse when standing)
- urinary dysfunction (retention, incontinence, frequency)
- bowel dysfunction

Consider requesting patient to complete validated questionnaire prior to clinic consultation, such as ICIQ-SF for incontinence, and bladder diary.

PATIENT EXAMINATION

Examination of the abdomen to evaluate for organomegaly, scars or palpable bladder

Pelvic examination of the patient is essential and therefore request female chaperone be present.

Undertake pelvic examination in standing, lithotomy and left lateral position (Sim's speculum):

- retract anterior wall to visualise posterior compartment prolapse
- retract posterior wall to demonstrate anterior / middle compartment prolapse
- undertake cough test for SUI

Perform urinalysis (send MSU for culture as appropriate), record PVR.

Consider MRI scan for select cases or surgical planning.

MANAGEMENT

CONSERVATIVE

Counsel patient carefully in presence of community continence nurse.

Consider weight loss, moderate exercise, treating cough / constipation and supervised PFMT, treat vaginal atrophy where appropriate.

Vaginal pessary is an option – individually fitted and changed every 3–6 months, where examination must be undertaken to check for vaginal erosion or ulceration.

SURGICAL

Prior to active intervention, the patient should be discussed at the local pelvic floor MDT.

There are many different approaches depending on the underlying POP pathology.

For uterine prolapse consider hysterectomy (abdominal / vaginal) or sacro-hysteropexy if the patient wishes to preserve their uterus.

Repair may be with primary colposuspension or with absorbable buttress sutures and mesh insertion.

BLADDER DYSFUNCTION AND GYNAECOLOGICAL ASPECTS OF UROLOGY MCQS

1. Where do the fibres of the pudendal nerve originate from?
   A) ventromedial nucleus
   B) Barrington's nucleus
   C) Onuf's nucleus
   D) Clarke's nucleus
   E) periaqueductal gray

2. Below which spinal level is autonomic dysreflexia less likely to occur?
   A) T4
   B) T6
   C) T8
   D) T10
   E) T12

3. What is the correct minimum PFMT regime as recommended by NICE (2019)?
   A) ≥ 6 contractions, twice daily
   B) ≥ 8 contractions, twice daily
   C) ≥ 4 contractions, three times daily
   D) ≥ 6 contractions, three times daily
   E) ≥ 8 contractions, three times daily

4. Which of the following is not a contraindication to anticholinergic medication?
   A) congestive heart failure
   B) pyloric stenosis
   C) severe ulcerative colitis
   D) urinary retention
   E) intestinal atony

5. Which muscarinic receptors does tolterodine primarily block?
   A) M1
   B) M2
   C) M3
   D) M2 and M3
   E) none of the above

6. What is the approximate half-life of solifenacin?
   A) 15–30 hours
   B) 30–45 hours
   C) 45–60 hours
   D) 60–75 hours
   E) 75–90 hours

7. What is the approximate half-life of mirabegron?
   A) 10 hours
   B) 20 hours
   C) 30 hours
   D) 40 hours
   E) 50 hours

8. Which statement regarding the DIGNITY study for BOTOX is false?
   A) the trigone was not injected
   B) both MS and SCI patients benefited
   C) only neuropathic patients were included
   D) no difference in efficacy was noted between 100units and 200units dose
   E) the end-point follow up was after 6 weeks

9. If VLPP is noted to be < 60cm H_2O during UDS assessment for SUI, what is the most likely underlying problem?
   A) detrusor hyperreflexia
   B) anatomical cause
   C) urethral hypermobility
   D) hypotonic detrusor muscle
   E) intrinsic sphincter deficiency

10. Which of the following statements regarding duloxetine is false?
    A) inhibits reuptake of noradrenaline
    B) it can be prescribed for a patient also taking warfarin
    C) yawning is a common side effect
    D) severe diarrhoea and vomiting should prompt immediate cessation
    E) it can be prescribed in pregnancy

11. What pressure should the pressure regulating balloon be set at in the AUS device?
    A) 41–50cm H_2O
    B) 51–60cm H_2O
    C) 61–70cm H_2O
    D) 71–80cm H_2O
    E) 81–90cm H_2O

12. A patient who has undergone UDS has a Q_{max} of 12mL/s and $P_{det}Q_{max}$ of 77cm H_2O. What is the correct value of their bladder outlet obstruction index?
    A) 53
    B) 41
    C) 89
    D) 101
    E) 65

13. What is the approximate adherence rate after 12 months for patients starting anticholinergic medication?
    A) 20–25%
    B) 30–35%
    C) 40–45%
    D) 50–55%
    E) 60–65%

14. Which statement is correct regarding the motor innervation of the bladder is true?
    A) post-ganglionic parasympathetic nuclei are located at S2–4
    B) the predominant effect of the sympathetic nerves is parasympathetic inhibition
    C) parasympathetic nerves provide cholinergic inhibitory input to the detrusor
    D) parasympathetic nerves provide excitatory input to the bladder neck
    E) the nuclei of the pre-ganglionic sympathetic nerves lie in the hypogastric plexus

15. A patient who has undergone UDS has a Q_{max} of 12mL/s and $P_{det}Q_{max}$ of 77cm H_2O. What is the correct value of their bladder contractility index?
    A) 17
    B) 101
    C) 137
    D) 113
    E) 41

16. Which nerve roots does the bulbocavernous reflex test?
    A) T10 – S2
    B) T12 – S2
    C) T12 – S4
    D) S2 – S4
    E) S1 – S2

17. Which of the following statements regarding the urethral sphincter innervation is false?
    A) perineal branch of pudendal nerve is for motor input
    B) relaxation is mediated by nitric oxide
    C) Onuf's nucleus is located in the ventral part of the anterior horn of the sacral cord
    D) the intrinsic sphincter is absent anteriorly
    E) the skeletal muscle component is the outermost layer

18. Where is the periaqueductal gray matter located?
    A) within tegmentum of midbrain
    B) within corpora quadrigemina around the cerebral aqueduct
    C) within the substancia nigra
    D) within the reticular formation
    E) within the crus cerebri

19. Which of the following statements regarding mirabegron is true?
    A) it inhibits adenylyl cyclase
    B) it is metabolised by the kidneys and excreted in the urine
    C) angioedema is a common side effect
    D) it is safe in breast feeding
    E) it promotes cAMP stimulation

20. What is the most common type of cancer found in female urethral diverticulum?
    A) transitional cell carcinoma
    B) adenocarcinoma
    C) squamous cell carcinoma
    D) sarcoma
    E) mucinous cell carcinoma

REFERENCES

1. Nayar C, Kalsi V, Hamid R et al. (2018) In: Arya M, Shergill IS, Fernando HS, et al. Viva Practice for the FRCS (Urol) and Postgraduate Urology Examinations, CRC Press, London
2. Chai TC, Steers WD, (1996). Neurophysiology of micturition and continence. *Urologic Clinics*, 23(2), 221–236.
3. Reynard J, Brewster S, Biers S (2013) Neuropathic bladder. In: Oxford Handbook of Urology 3rd Edition, Oxford University Press, Oxford.
4. Park JM, Bloom DA, McGuire EJ. (1997). The guarding reflex revisited. *British journal of urology*, 80(6), 940–945.
5. Blok B, Castro-Diaz D, Del Popolo G, et al. (2020) EAU Guidelines: Neuro-urology. Available at: https://uroweb.org/guideline/neuro-urology/#3 [last accessed on 10 June 2020]
6. Fowler CJ. (1999). Neurological disorders of micturition and their treatment. *Brain*, 122(7), 1213–1231.
7. Stocchi F, Carbone A, Inghilleri M, et al. (1997) Urodynamic and neurophysiological evaluation in Parkinson's disease and multiple system atrophy. *Journal of Neurology, Neurosurgery & Psychiatry*, 62(5), 507–511.
8. Karlsson AK. (1999). Autonomic dysreflexia. *Spinal cord*, 37(6), 383–391.
9. Krassioukov A, Warburton DE, Teasell R, et al. (2009) A systematic review of the management of autonomic dysreflexia after spinal cord injury. *Archives of physical medicine and rehabilitation*, 90(4), 682–695.
10. From British Association of Urological Surgeons. Available at: https://www.baus.org.uk/_userfiles/pages/files/Patients/Leaflets/ICIQ-UI.pdf [last accessed 10 June 2020]
11. Chevalier F, Fernandez-Lao C, Cuesta-Vargas AI. (2014) Normal reference values of strength in pelvic floor muscle of women: a descriptive and inferential study. *BMC women's health*, 14(1), 143.
12. NICE (2019) Guidelines: Urinary incontinence and pelvic organ prolapse in women: management. Available at: https://www.nice.org.uk/guidance/ng123/resources/urinary-incontinence-and-pelvic-organ-prolapse-in-women-management-pdf-66141657205189 [last accessed 10 June 2020]
13. Novara G, Galfano A, Secco S, et al. (2008) A systematic review and meta-analysis of randomized controlled trials with antimuscarinic drugs for overactive bladder. *European urology*, 54(4), 740–764.
14. Reynolds WS, McPheeters M, Blume J, et al. (2015) Comparative effectiveness of anticholinergic therapy for overactive bladder in women: a systematic review and meta-analysis. *Obstetrics & Gynecology*, 125(6), 1423–1432.

15. Richardson K, Fox C, Maidment I, et al. (2018) Anticholinergic drugs and risk of dementia: case-control study. *bmj*, *361*, k1315.
16. Gray SL, Anderson ML, Dublin S, et al. (2015) Cumulative use of strong anticholinergics and incident dementia: a prospective cohort study. *JAMA internal medicine*, *175*(3), 401–407.
17. Chapple CR, Cardozo L, Nitti VW, et al. (2014) Mirabegron in overactive bladder: a review of efficacy, safety, and tolerability. *Neurourology and urodynamics*, *33*(1), 17–30.
18. Cruz F, Herschorn S, Aliotta P, et al. (2011) Efficacy and safety of onabotulinumtoxinA in patients with urinary incontinence due to neurogenic detrusor overactivity: a randomised, double-blind, placebo-controlled trial. *European urology*, *60*(4), 742–750.
19. Nitti VW, Dmochowski R, Herschorn S, et al. (2013) OnabotulinumtoxinA for the treatment of patients with overactive bladder and urinary incontinence: results of a phase 3, randomized, placebo controlled trial. *The Journal of urology*, *189*(6), 2186–2193.
20. Blaivas JG, Olsson CA. (1988) Stress incontinence: classification and surgical approach. *The Journal of urology*, *139*(4), 727–731.
21. Jost W, Marsalek P. (2004) Duloxetine: mechanism of action at the lower urinary tract and Onuf's nucleus. *Clinical Autonomic Research*, *14*(4), 220–227.
22. Brubaker L, Cundiff GW, Fine P, et al. (2006) Abdominal sacrocolpopexy with Burch colposuspension to reduce urinary stress incontinence. *New England Journal of Medicine*, *354*(15), 1557–1566.
23. Lim CS, Abrams P. (1995) The Abrams-Griffiths nomogram. *World journal of urology*, *13*(1), 34–39.
24. Blaivas JG, Groutz A. (2000) Bladder outlet obstruction nomogram for women with lower urinary tract symptomatology. *Neurourology and Urodynamics: Official Journal of the International Continence Society*, *19*(5), 553–564.
25. Romanzi LJ, Groutz A, Blaivas JG. (2000). Urethral diverticulum in women: diverse presentations resulting in diagnostic delay and mismanagement. *The Journal of urology*, *164*(2), 428–433.
26. Wall LL. (2006) Obstetric vesicovaginal fistula as an international public-health problem. *The Lancet*, *368*(9542), 1201–1209.
27. Stamatakos M, Sargedi C, Stasinou T, (2014). Vesicovaginal fistula: diagnosis and management. *Indian Journal of Surgery*, *76*(2), 131–136.
28. Persu C, Chapple CR, Cauni V, et al. (2011) Pelvic Organ Prolapse Quantification System (POP-Q)–a new era in pelvic prolapse staging. *Journal of medicine and life*, *4*(1), 75.

STATION 8
BPH AND ANDROLOGY

PROSTATE ANATOMY AND DEVELOPMENT

EJACULATORY DISORDERS

ERECTILE DYSFUNCTION

HYPOGONADISM

LUTS

MALE INFERTILITY

PEYRONIE'S DISEASE

TREATMENT OF BPH

VARICOCOELE

CONTENTS

PROSTATE ANATOMY & DEVELOPMENT — **227**
   ARTERIAL SUPPLY — 227
   VENOUS DRAINAGE — 227
   LYMPH DRAINAGE — 228
   EMBRYOLOGY OF PROSTATE — 228
   ZONAL ANATOMY — 228
   PHYSIOLOGY OF BPH — 230
     ROLE OF ANDROGENS IN BPH — 230

EJACULATORY DISORDERS — **232**
   RETROGRADE EJACULATION — 232
     AETIOLOGY — 232
     DIAGNOSTIC EVALUATION — 232
     MANAGEMENT — 232
   PREMATURE EJACULATION — 233
     AETIOLOGY — 233
     DIAGNOSTIC EVALUATION — 233
     MANAGEMENT — 234
   ANEJACULATION — 234
     VASECTOMY — 234
     VASECTOMY REVERSAL — 235

ERECTILE DYSFUNCTION — **237**
   PENILE ANATOMY — 237
     ARTERIAL SUPPLY — 237
     VENOUS DRAINAGE — 237
     INNERVATION — 238
     CROSS-SECTIONAL VIEW — 238
   PHYSIOLOGY OF ERECTION — 239
     CAVERNOSAL SMOOTH MUSCLE — 240
     EJACULATION — 241
     EPIDEMIOLOGY — 242
     AETIOLOGY — 242
   DIAGNOSTIC EVALUATION — 243

PATIENT HISTORY	243
PATIENT EXAMINATION	245
BASELINE INVESTIGATIONS	245
RIGISCAN DEVICE	246
PENILE COLOUR DOPPLER	246
CAVERNOSOGRAPHY	246
MANAGEMENT	247
CONSERVATIVE	247
PHOSPHODIESTERASE TYPE-5 INHIBITORS (1ST LINE)	247
VACUUM ERECTION DEVICE (2ND LINE)	249
INTRA-CAVERNOSAL INJECTIONS (2ND LINE)	250
INTRA-URETHRAL ALPROSTADIL (MUSE) (2ND LINE)	250
TOPICAL ALPROSTADIL (2ND LINE)	250
SHOCKWAVE LITHOTRIPSY	250
PENILE PROSTHESES (3RD LINE)	250
ED POST RADICAL PROSTATECTOMY	251
HYPOGONADISM	**252**
PATHOPHYSIOLOGY	252
DIAGNOSTIC EVALUATION	252
PATIENT HISTORY	252
PATIENT EXAMINATION	252
BASELINE INVESTIGATIONS	253
SHBG	253
MANAGEMENT	253
LUTS DIAGNOSTIC EVALUATION	**255**
PATIENT HISTORY	255
PATIENT EXAMINATION	257
BASELINE INVESTIGATIONS	257
UROFLOWMETRY	259
EPIDEMIOLOGY	259
INFERTILITY	**260**
MALE REPRODUCTIVE PHYSIOLOGY	260
SPERMATOGENESIS	260

DEFINITIONS	261
EPIDEMIOLOGY	262
SEMEN CHARACTERISTICS	262
AETIOLOGY	263
DIAGNOSTIC EVALUATION	264
PATIENT HISTORY	264
PATIENT EXAMINATION	264
INVESTIGATIONS	265
BASELINE	265
IMAGING	265
VASOGRAPHY	266
TESTICULAR BIOPSY	266
OLIGOSPERMIA	267
AZOOSPERMIA	267
INVESTIGATIONS	267
MANAGEMENT	268
Y MICRO-DELETION	269
MALE ASSISTED CONCEPTION	270
INTRAUTERINE INSEMINATION (IUI)	270
IVF AND ICSI	270
SPERM RETRIEVAL TECHNIQUES	271
PEYRONIE'S DISEASE	**272**
EPIDEMIOLOGY	272
AETIOLOGY	272
RISK FACTORS	273
DIAGNOSTIC EVALUATION	273
PATIENT HISTORY	273
PATIENT EXAMINATION	274
MANAGEMENT	274
CONSERVATIVE	274
MEDICAL	274
SURGICAL	276
PD SURGERY ALGORITHM	278
TREATMENT OF BPH	**279**

WATCHFUL WAITING	279
MEDICAL THERAPY	279
α-1 ADRENORECEPTOR ANTAGONISTS	279
5α-REDUCTASE INHIBITORS	280
COMBINATION THERAPY	282
PHYTOTHERAPY	284
TURP	284
HOLEP	285
UROLIFT™	286
ACUTE URINARY RETENTION	286
VARICOCOELE	**289**
EPIDEMIOLOGY	289
AETIOLOGY	289
CLASSIFICATION	289
DIAGNOSTIC EVALUATION	290
MANAGEMENT	290
REFERENCES	**292**
ANDROLOGY AND BPH MCQS	**294**

PROSTATE ANATOMY & DEVELOPMENT

ARTERIAL SUPPLY

Internal iliac artery

→ anterior branch → inferior vesical artery → branches to the prostate

From the urethral group of arteries arise *Flock's* (1 and 11 o'clock) and *Badenoch's* (5 and 7 o'clock) arteries to supply the transitional zone of the prostate.

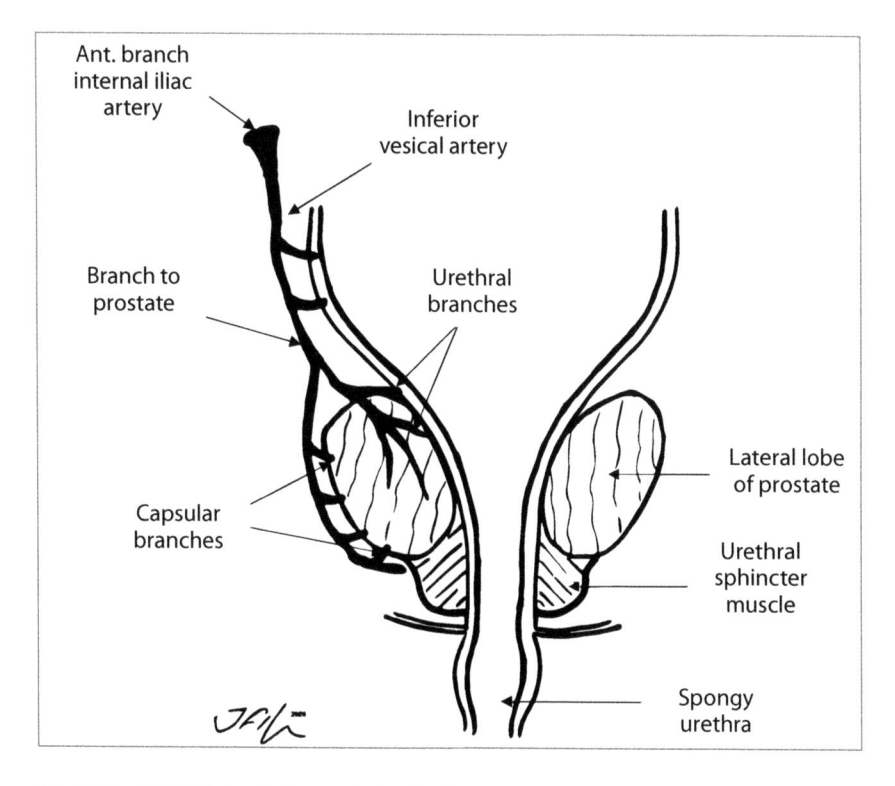

Image 1 – Arterial supply to prostate gland

VENOUS DRAINAGE

Via the peri-prostatic venous plexus (which also receives the deep dorsal vein of the penis)

→ drains into internal iliac vein → ipsilateral common iliac vein

LYMPH DRAINAGE

Lymphatic drainage of the prostate is mainly to the obturator nodes and subsequently to the internal iliac chain.

There is also lymphatic communication with the external iliac, presacral, and the para-aortic lymph nodes.

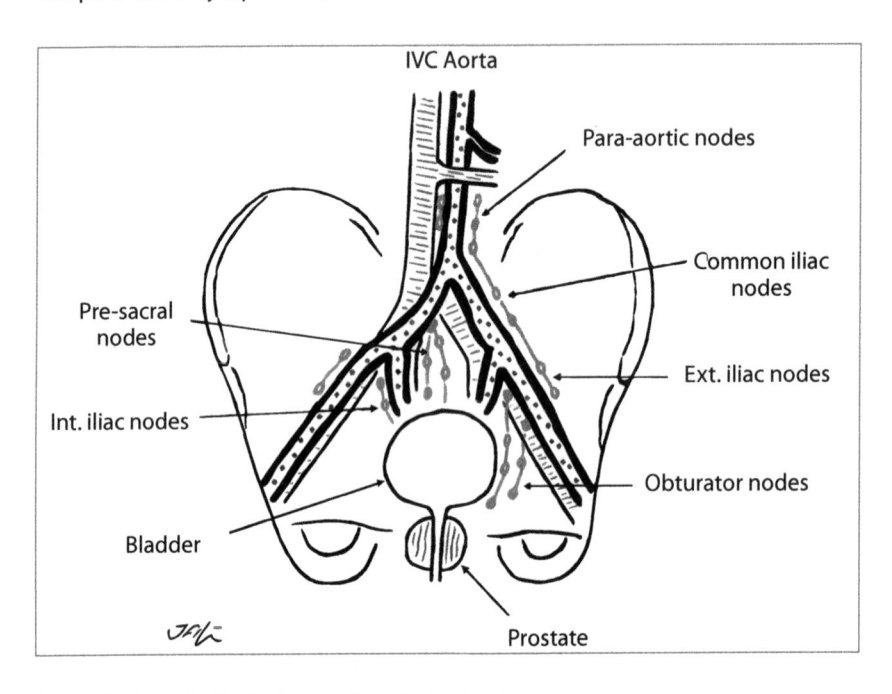

Image 2 – Lymphatic drainage of prostate gland

EMBRYOLOGY OF PROSTATE

Dual embryological origin – central zone derived from mesonephric duct, rest of prostate from the urogenital sinus

At approximately 16 weeks gestation it arises under direct influence of 5-DHT.

ZONAL ANATOMY

McNeal described zones of the prostate from pathology specimens, however the prostate is often described anatomically using lobes (anterior, median, posterior and 2 lateral). [1] [Table 1]

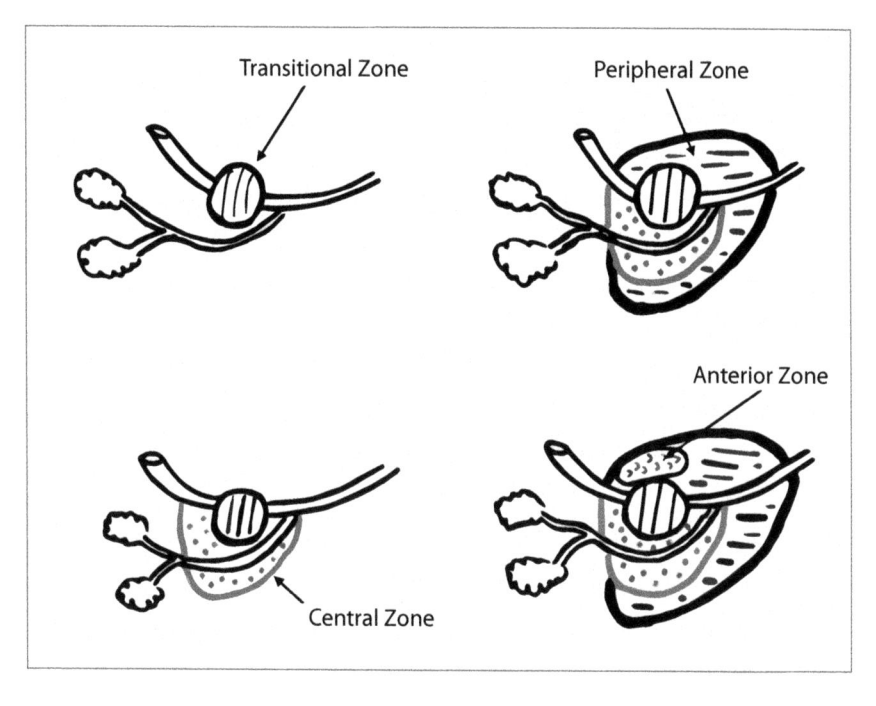

Image 3 – Zonal anatomy of prostate gland

Table 1 – McNeal's zones of the prostate

McNeal Zone		Description
Peripheral zone	≤ 70% of glandular tissues	Site of origin for 70–80% of prostate cancers
Central zone	25% of glandular tissue	Zone surrounding ejaculatory ducts, < 5% cancers originate here.
Transition zone	10% of glandular tissue	Site of origin of BPH tissue changes
Anterior fibro-muscular stroma	Approximately 5%	no glandular components, composed of muscle and fibrous tissue

PHYSIOLOGY OF BPH

Benign prostatic *enlargement* (BPE) is characterised by an increase in epithelial and stromal cell numbers in the peri-urethral area of the prostate (i.e. transition zone).

Benign prostatic *hyperplasia* (BPH) properly describes the histological findings of suspected BPE.

Combination of increased cell proliferation (early phase) and reduction in apoptosis (latter phase)

In established BPH, cell proliferation slows down and programmed cell death is impaired.

Normal stromal tissue has substantial smooth muscle component (~50%), however in BPH the proportion of this is less (~25%).

The symptoms and effects of BPE are caused by two main components:

- *static*, mediated by volume effect of BPE
- *dynamic*, due to α-adrenoreceptor mediated prostatic smooth muscle contraction

This is the rationale for α-adrenoreceptor blocker treatment (e.g. tamsulosin).

ROLE OF ANDROGENS IN BPH

Testosterone can bind to androgen receptor directly, or may be converted to a more potent form called dihydrotestosterone (DHT)

This conversion is mediated by the enzyme 5α-reductase (5AR) which can be:

- *type-1* (extra-prostatic, in liver and skin) or
- *type-2* (found exclusively on nuclear membrane of stromal cells (not epithelial cells)

Finasteride inhibits type-2 only, reducing serum DHT by 70% and prostatic DHT by 80%. [2]

Dutasteride inhibits both type-1 and 2, reducing serum DHT by 95% and prostatic DHT by 94%. [3]

This difference in their respective reductions of DHT however does not translate into a known difference in their clinical efficacies.

Testosterone diffuses into prostate stromal and epithelial cells:

- within epithelial cells it binds directly to androgen receptor (AR)
- within stromal cell the majority binds to type II (5AR), is converted to DHT which binds to the androgen receptor (with greater affinity and potency)

The AR / testosterone or AR / DHT complexes bind in nucleus to induce transcription of androgen-dependent genes and protein synthesis. [Figure 1]

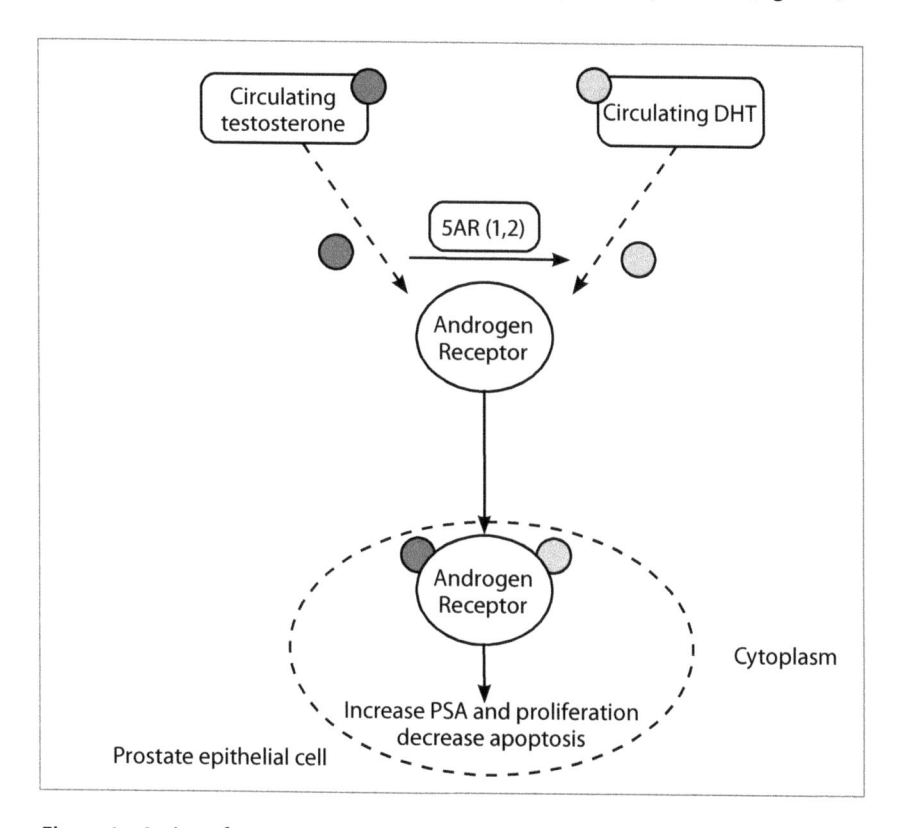

Figure 1 – Action of testosterone and DHT in prostate epithelial cell

EJACULATORY DISORDERS

RETROGRADE EJACULATION

Retrograde ejaculation (RE) involves failure of bladder neck contraction causing retrograde flow of sperm into bladder on ejaculation.

AETIOLOGY

Acquired causes of RE include:
- iatrogenic anatomical disruption, e.g. TURP, BNI
- drugs, e.g. α-blockers (reversible), SSRIs, risperidone
- neurological, e.g. diabetic neuropathy, retro-peritoneal dissection

Congenital causes of RE include spina bifida.

DIAGNOSTIC EVALUATION

The key factors in the patient history include:
- dry ejaculate at orgasm followed by cloudy urine
- assess for risk factors as listed above (drugs, previous surgery)
- may present to the clinician as infertility

Patient examination may be unremarkable.

Perform *semen analysis* (low ejaculate volume < 1mL).

A post-orgasm urine examination reveals sperm in specimen to confirm the diagnosis.

MANAGEMENT

Treatment is only needed if patient is wishing to preserve natural fertility.

Reversible causes (such as α-blockers) should be addressed.

Medical Treatment

Medication can be used to try and close the bladder neck.

Sympathomimetics (α-adrenergics) such as pseudoephedrine can be given 7–10 days prior to planned ejaculation (often in view of female ovulation time).

Imipramine (tri-cyclic anti-depressant) may also be used.

Sperm Retrieval

If medical therapy fails, sperm can be retrieved from alkalinised post-ejaculate urine (acidic urine is thought to be spermicidal).

Patient is to take sodium bicarbonate orally the night before and morning of producing sample.

Patient empties bladder, then masturbates and after a post-ejaculation urine sample is collected and delivered to the laboratory.

The lab will centrifuge the sample – retrieved sperm can also be used for IVF or IUI.

PREMATURE EJACULATION

There is no validated or accurate definition for diagnosing premature ejaculation (PrE).

International Society for Sexual Medicine proposes time limit < 1 minute from vaginal penetration. [4]

- inability to delay ejaculation
- negative personal consequences / low satisfaction with sexual relationship

AETIOLOGY

Organic – penile hyper-sensitivity, central serotonin receptor abnormalities

Psychogenic

DIAGNOSTIC EVALUATION

The key factors in the patient history include:

- is problem lifelong or acquired (precipitating factor)
- impact on patient QOL / relationships / mood
- estimated time from penetration to ejaculation

Patient examination is likely to be unremarkable in relation to PrE, ensure no genitalia abnormality.

Do not routinely undertake laboratory tests.

MANAGEMENT

Behavioural
1. Master's and Johnson's squeeze technique
2. Seman's stop-start technique

Pharmacological

SSRIs are the only NICE approved treatment for PrE (eg. citalopram, paroxetine), these should be taken on demand several hours prior to intercourse.

(Serotonin is inhibitory neurotransmitter in control of ejaculation.)

Topical lidocaine is an option, however may lead to penile hypo-aesthesia or vaginal numbness.

ANEJACULATION

The complete absence of antegrade / retrograde ejaculation is termed anejaculation.

This condition can be caused by:
- spinal cord injury
- congenital bilateral absence of vas deferens (CBAVD) seen in CF
- retro-peritoneal lymph node dissection

Semen can be obtained using a Seager electro-ejaculator (rectal probe stimulation) or retrieval can be undertaken to be used for IVF and IUI.

VASECTOMY

A patient requesting vasectomy should be seen in the routine general urology clinic.

Assess for key factors in the *patient history*:
- current family and future family plans
- awareness of alternative methods of contraception for himself and partner
- age

- previous scrotal surgery (might make surgery under local anaesthesia challenging)

Ensure that on *patient examination* in clinic you can feel both vas easily.

If patient is keen to proceed, the following risks / side effects must be discussed:
- early failure rate (1 in 250)
- late failure rate (1 in 2000) due to re-canalisation
- chronic testicular pain (5%)
- bruising / haematoma requiring drainage / infection
- not reversible on the NHS

After vasectomy patient must continue to use barrier contraception.

Sperm needs to be cleared by normal ejaculation (20–30 ejaculations required).

≥ 12 weeks after vasectomy patient must have semen analysis – a single azoospermic sample after this timeframe is sufficient to give patient "all clear" to have unprotected sex. [5]

For those not azoospermic at first test sample, 95% will be at repeat sampling 6 weeks later.

Special clearance can be given 28 weeks post-vasectomy, provided < 10^5 / mL of non-motile sperm.

VASECTOMY REVERSAL

Approximately 6% of men will request a reversal of vasectomy (e.g. new partner). [6]

The surgery requires micro-apposition of the vas ends:
- multi-layer vaso-vasostomy
- single-layer vaso-vasostomy
- inguinal vaso-vasostomy (eg. if vas obstructed within inguinal canal from hernia repair)
- epididymo-vaso-vasostomy (EVV)

The key principle is precise end approximation (prevent sperm leakage and granuloma formation) and non-tension (compromise blood supply).

A sample of sperm fluid should be taken from the proximal vas and analysed.

EVV may be required if secondary obstruction at level of epididymis (resulting in low volume or devoid of sperm).

Success rates depend on time interval since vasectomy was performed. [Table 2]

Table 2 – Patency and pregnancy rates categorised by time since vasectomy [7]

Time from vasectomy (years)	Patency rate (%)	Pregnancy rate (%)
< 3	97	76
3–8	88	53
9–14	79	44
≥ 15	71	30

If reversal is not successful, patient can alternatively undergo sperm retrieval procedure.

NHS offers ≤ 3 cycles of IVF according to access criteria as per NICE (although local CCGs may have their own additional criteria): [8]

- women < 40 years who have not conceived after 2 years of regular unprotected sex
- women 40–42 years who have not conceived after 2 years of regular unprotected sex, provided they have not had IVF cycle before (offer 1 cycle)

ERECTILE DYSFUNCTION

PENILE ANATOMY

ARTERIAL SUPPLY

Internal iliac artery (ant. branch) → internal pudendal artery → common penile artery (main supply)

Accessory supply may derive from branches of external iliac, obturator, vesical and femoral artery.

The main branches of the common penile artery:
- *cavernous*: involved in tumescence of corpora cavernosa (via helicine branches, which become dilated and straight during erection)
- *dorsal*: provides engorgement of penis during erection
- *bulbar*: to supply bulb and corpus spongiosum

VENOUS DRAINAGE

Venous drainage from the three corpora:
- originate in venules, travel between tunica and peripheral sinusoids
- form the sub-tunical venular plexus before exiting as emissary veins

Outside the tunica albuginea, the venous drainage is dependent on the area of drainage:

Skin: multiple superficial veins unite near root of penis
 → to form superficial dorsal vein
  → drains into saphenous veins

Corpora: the emissary veins drain into deep dorsal vein (dorsally), circumflex vein (laterally) and peri-urethral veins (ventrally).

proximal corpora cavernosa drains into cavernous and crural veins

distal 2 / 3 corpora → deep dorsal vein → drains into peri-prostatic venous plexus

INNERVATION

Autonomic

Sympathetic nerves (T11–L2) and para-sympathetic nerves (S2–4) join to form pelvic plexus.

Cavernosal nerves are branches of pelvic plexus that innervate penis:
- parasympathetic causes erection
- sympathetic causes ejaculation and detumescence

Somatic

Sensory (afferent) information travels via dorsal penile and pudendal nerves to enter cord S2–4.

Onuf's nucleus (S2–4) is somatic centre for efferent innervation of ischio- and bulbo-cavernous muscles of the penis.

CROSS-SECTIONAL VIEW

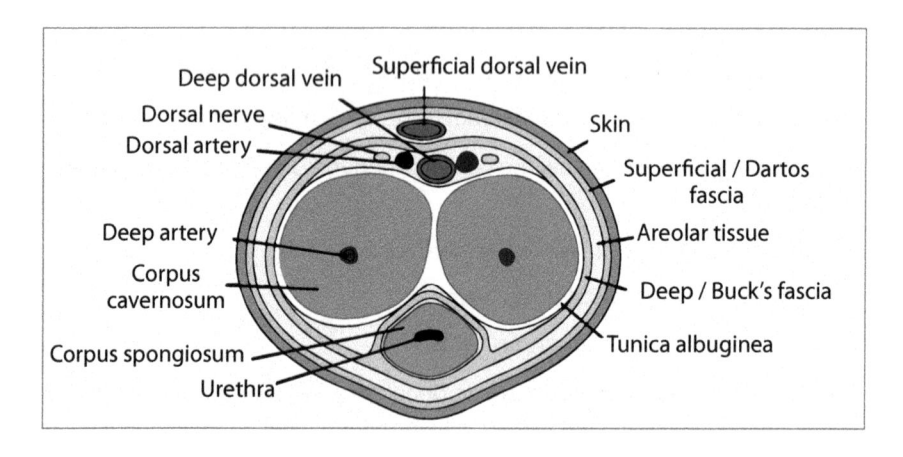

Image 4 – Cross-sectional anatomical view of penis [9]

Bucks fascia fuses with tunica albuginea proximally.

Dartos fascia in continuity with Scarpa's fascia

All the urethra has transitional cell epithelium, except fossa navicularis which has squamous.

PHYSIOLOGY OF ERECTION

In the flaccid state, the smooth muscle of the arteriolar walls is tonically contracted, allowing only small amount of arterial flow into cavernous spaces.

Subsequently audio / tactile / visual stimuli create neuroendocrine signals from the brain.

These activate the autonomic nuclei of the spinal erection centre (T11–L2) and (S2–4).

Signals are conveyed via cavernosal nerve to erectile tissue of corpora cavernosa, releasing neurotransmitters from the cavernous nerve terminals.

This results in smooth muscle relaxation, activating the *veno-occlusive mechanism* and triggering the following sequence of events:

- dilatation of arterioles / arteries by increased blood flow
- trapping of incoming blood by expanding sinusoids
- compression of sub-tunical venular plexuses (reduces venous outflow)
- stretching tunica to capacity which encloses emissary veins (reduces venous outflow)
- rise in intra-cavernous pressure (approx. 100mmHg) – *full erection* phase
- further pressure rise due to ischio-cavernous muscle contraction – *rigid erection* phase

There are five distinct phases of penile erection that have been demonstrated.

Detumescence has initial, slow and fast phases.

Table 3 – Phases of erection

Phase	Term (Phase)	Description
0	Flaccid	Cavernosal muscle contracted
		Sinusoids empty
		Minimal arterial flow
1	Latent (filling)	Increased pudendal artery flow (peak flow ~ 25mL / min at end of latent phase)
		Penile elongation
2	Tumescent	Rising intra-cavernosal pressure
		Erection forming
3	Full erection	Increased cavernosal pressure
		Penis becomes full erect
4	Rigid erection	Further increases in pressure (peak intra-corporeal pressure, minimal blood flow)
		Ischio-cavernous muscle contraction
5	Detumescent	Sympathetic discharge continues after ejaculation
		Smooth muscle contraction / vasoconstriction
		Reduced arterial flow, blood out from sinusoidal spaces

CAVERNOSAL SMOOTH MUSCLE

Nitric oxide (NO)

Vaso-active intestinal peptide (VIP) → Decrease in Calcium → RELAXATION (erection)

Prostaglandin E_1 (PGE_1)

Following ejaculation, vasocontriction (by sympathetic activity, endothelin, PGF_2, cGMP breakdown) causes detumescence

Noradrenaline released from sympathetic nerve terminals act on smooth muscle α-1 adrenoreceptors to raise intra-cellular calcium helping maintain flaccidity

Noradrenaline (NA)

Endothelin-1 ➔ Increased calcium sensitivity ➔ CONTRACTION (flaccidity)

Prostaglandin F_2 (PGF_2)

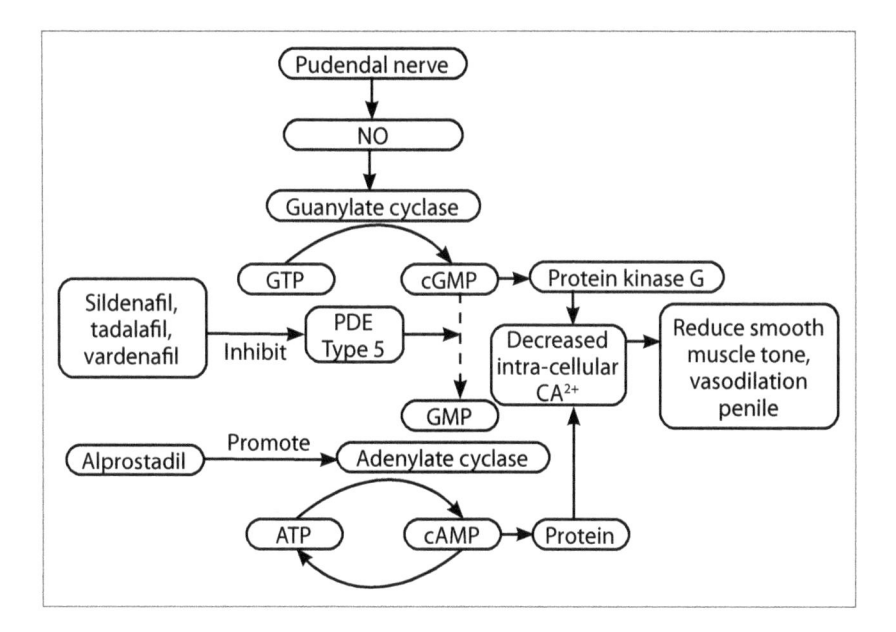

Figure 2 – Secondary messenger pathways involved in erection

EJACULATION

Stimulation sends sensory information via pudendal nerve to lumbar sympathetic nuclei.

Sympathetic efferent signs via hypogastric nerve causing:
- contraction of smooth muscle of epididymis, vas deferent, secretory glands
- propelling spermatozoa and glandular secretions into prostatic urethra
- closure of internal urethral sphincter and relaxation of extrinsic sphincter
- rhythmic contraction of bulbo-cavernous muscle for emission of ejaculate

Volume of ejaculate is 2–5mL

Contribution is prostatic (first) (0.5mL), sperm (next), then seminal vesicle (2mL)

EPIDEMIOLOGY

Incidence increases with age – complete erectile dysfunction (ED) in 70s (15%) and 80s (30–40%)

Mild ED present in at least 20% of aged 30–80years

ED shares common risk factors for cardio-vascular disease (they have a bi-directional relationship).

AETIOLOGY

ED divided into primary psychogenic vs. primary organic causes (although commonly mixed)

ED has a strong association with age, diabetic duration and control (ED can be first presenting symptom of diabetes in 20%), BMI.

An organic cause is more likely in the following scenarios:
- gradual onset (unless cause is obvious such as trauma / pelvic surgery)
- loss of spontaneous (morning) erections as well
- libido is intact with normal ejaculatory function
- existing medical factors and older age groups

Sexual history should be taken bearing in mind all potential causes of ED (which is a symptom). [Table 4]

Table 4 – Categorised causes of erectile dysfunction

Cause	Examples of diseases
Vasculogenic	CVD, diabetes, hyper-lipidaemia, smoking
Neurogenic	CKD, SCI, CVA, MS, Parkinson's, Surgery / Radio-Tx to pelvis / prostate
Anatomical	Peyronie's, micropenis, phimosis
Hormonal	Hypogonadism, hypo-/hyper-thyroid, high prolactin, high-low cortisol
Drug-induced	SSRIs, tri-cyclics, anti-psychotics, alcohol, cocaine, β-blockers, thiazides
Trauma	Penile and pelvic fractures
Psychogenic	Anxiety, depression

Consistent evidence for association between LUTS / BPH and ED in older men

Simple modification of risk factors can improve ED, the most important factor associated with recovery of erections after RP is pre-operative potency.

DIAGNOSTIC EVALUATION

PATIENT HISTORY

Patient should ideally be seen in specialist andrology / sexual dysfunction clinic, in presence of partner and andrology specialist nurse.

A full sexual history should be taken, including enquiry regarding:
- duration of ED
- morning erections present / absent
- situational: present on masturbation, vary depending on partner
- risk factors
- full drug history / alcohol / smoking
- psychosocial factors
- presence of LUTS

A validated questionnaire can be used to assess the severity of the ED.

These are helpful in assessing domains of sexual function as well as impact of treatment.

The International Index of Erectile Function (IIEF) or the shorter version (IIEF-5) can be used and relates to the last 6 months: [10]

1	How do you rate your confidence that you could get and keep an erection	Very Low	Low	Moderate	High	Very High
		1	2	3	4	5
2	When you had erections with sexual stimulation, how often were your erections hard enough for penetration	Almost never/ never	A few times (much less than half the time)	Sometimes (about half the time)	Most times (much more than half the time)	Almost always/ always
		1	2	3	4	5
3	During sexual intercourse, how often were you able to maintain your erection after you had penetrated (entered) your partner?	Almost never/ never	A few times (much less than half the time)	Sometimes (about half the time)	Most times (much more than half the time)	Almost always/ always
		1	2	3	4	5
4	During sexual intercourse, how difficult was it to maintain your erection to completion of intercourse	Extremely difficult	Very difficult	Difficult	Slightly difficult	Not difficult
		1	2	3	4	5
5	When you attempted sexual intercourse, how often was it satisfactory for you?	Almost never/ never	A few times (much less than half the time)	Sometimes (about half the time)	Most times (much more than half the time)	Almost always/ always
		1	2	3	4	5

Image 5 – IIEF-5 questionnaire [10]

The overall score allows the severity of ED to be assessed objectively:

Table 5 – Score categories for IIEF-5 questionnaire

Score	Severity
1–7	Severe
8–11	Moderate
12–16	Mild to moderate
17–21	Mild
22–25	No ED

PATIENT EXAMINATION

A full physical examination is mandatory in the presence of a chaperone.

The following organ systems should be assessed:
- cardiovascular: measure BP, HR and BMI / waist circumference
- genitalia: size of testes, phimosis, evidence of Peyronie's
- DRE: assess for BPH or PCa
- neuro: (bulbo-cavernosus reflex test S2 – S4 integrity, squeeze glans → anal contraction)
- secondary sexual characteristic

BASELINE INVESTIGATIONS

Baseline investigations will depend on the history and examination of the patient.

Blood tests that should be considered include:
- fasting glucose and lipid profile
- serum (free) early morning testosterone (if low then perform LH, FSH, SHBG)
- prolactin
- PSA (if abnormal DRE)

Most referred patients with ED can be managed in the secondary care setting with no further tests than above.

Some patients may need specific diagnostic tests:

- primary ED (not caused by organic disease or psychogenic)
- young patients with pelvic / perineal trauma (may benefit from re-vascularisation)
- pre-implantation of penile prosthesis
- complex endocrine or psychiatric disorders
- penile deformities

RIGISCAN DEVICE

Nocturnal penile tumescence and rigidity testing (NPT)

Device containing two rings applied to penile tip and base, used to measure number / duration / rigidity of nocturnal erections

Helps the differentiation between psychogenic and organic pathology

Normal finding should be a 60% rigidity erection at the tip for ≥ 10 minutes.

PENILE COLOUR DOPPLER

Radiological investigation of choice if suspected underlying vascular cause for ED

Intra-cavernosal PGE1 injection is given to induce erection, the blood flow is then measured to diagnose *arteriogenic, veno-occlusive* or *mixed vasculogenic* ED.

Peak systolic velocity > 25–30cm / s (if lower than this value, suggests arteriogenic ED)

End diastolic velocity < 5cm / s (if higher than this, suggests veno-occlusive ED)

CAVERNOSOGRAPHY

A cavernosogram should only be performed in patients who are being considered for vascular reconstruction surgery.

Cavernosography requires artificial erection followed by injection of contrast into penis.

Flow is maintained throughout imaging to demonstrate any venous leaks.

Penile arteriography is rarely performed these days due to advent of penile prostheses, however contrast via pudendal artery is given before and after drug-induced erection.

Penile revascularisation surgery most commonly addresses internal pudendal artery stenosis.

MANAGEMENT

CONSERVATIVE

ED may be associated with modifiable or reversible risk factors (eg. Drugs, alcohol, high BMI).

These factors may be modified either before or during the time that specific therapies are used, including any relevant co-morbidities that need optimising.

Testosterone Supplementation

Testosterone deficiency may be primary (primary testicular failure) or secondary (low LH / FSH).

Testosterone supplementation (TS) is effective but should only be given once other endocrinological causes for low testosterone have been ruled out.

TS can be given oral / topical / IM with similar efficacy.

Prior to TS, you should perform DRE, PSA, haematocrit, liver profile and LFTs.

TS is contra-indicated in untreated PCa and unstable cardiac disease.

Oral agents are rapidly absorbed by the gut and broken down in first pass of liver metabolism (i.e. poorly effective), unless testosterone undecanoate is used which enters the lymphatic system.

Intra-muscular administration results in high peak / low trough levels (weekly or 6-weekly dosing) which can lead to mood swings, as well as pain at injection site.

PHOSPHODIESTERASE TYPE-5 INHIBITORS (1ST LINE)

Nitric oxide (NO) enters smooth muscle cell to activate soluble gunaylate cyclase (sGC), which catalyses GTP ➜ cGMP.

cGMP facilitates smooth muscle relaxation (reduction in intra-cellular calcium) for erection.

cGMP is terminated when metabolised to GMP (inactive) by PDE5 (ie. PDE5i prevent breakdown).

PDE5i therefore facilitate NO-induced smooth muscle relaxation by accumulation of cGMP.

Side effects of PDE5i include:
- headache, flushing, dizziness,
- nasal congestion
- back pain

PDE5i can be used in conjunction with TS.

Approximately 25% of patients do not respond to PDE5i – consider second line therapy.

Contra-indications

PDE5i are contra-indicated in patients taking nitrates – they result in cGMP accumulation and unpredictable falls in BP.

If PDE5i is taken, the nitrate must be with-held at least the length of the chosen PDE5 half-life.

PDE5i can be used with other anti-hypertensives with caution.

PDE5i should <u>not</u> be used if recent MI / stroke ≤ 6 months, severe heart failure, unstable angina or angina during intercourse.

Sildenafil (Viagra)

Sildenafil was the first PDE5i available on the market.

On demand medication with efficacy from 30 minutes after administration, which may be maintained for ≤ 12 hours.

Efficacy is reduced after heavy fatty meal due to delayed absorption.

Tadalafil (Cialis)

Efficacy is maintained for 36 hours, not affected by food (no reduced bio-availability).

Tadalafil is the only PDE5i available for daily dosing, therefore may be preferable for spontaneity.

Can be used to treat male LUTS (preferable option if ED co-existing with LUTS).

Vardenafil (Levitra)

Efficacy is reduced after heavy fatty meal due to delayed absorption.

Table 6 – Comparison of different PDE5i drugs

Drug	Dose (mg)	Modality	Half-life (hours)	Onset of action
Sildenafil	25, 50, 100	On demand	4–5	30 mins
Tadalafil	5, 10, 20	Daily (5) and on demand	17.5	30 mins (peak 120)
Vardenafil	5, 10, 20	On demand	4–5	30 mins

No trial has proven superior efficacy of any of the PDE5i drugs.

Drug choice will depend on patient preference regarding to number of intercourse per week, short vs. long lasting and side effects.

Medical failure should be confirmed only if patient fails to respond after ≥ 6 trials at maximum dosage, patient can then be offered daily dosing or 2nd line therapy.

IC_{50} (half maximal inhibitory concentration) refers to concentration of an antagonist that produces 50% of the maximum inhibitory effect of that antagonist (i.e. PDE5i is the antagonist).

Vardanafil's IC_{50} is 10x lower (i.e. the drug is more potent).

Eligibility

Patients can be offered PDE5i free on the NHS for following causes:
- Previous prostate surgery (e.g. TURP, RP)
- Nephrogenic (e.g. ESRF, dialysis)
- Neurogenic (e.g. diabetes, spinal cord injury)
- Severe psychological stress

VACUUM ERECTION DEVICE (2ND LINE)

Provide passive engorgement of corpora together with constrictor ring applied to base of penis

Satisfaction rates ≤ 90%, most who discontinue do so within first 3 months.

Contra-indicated in bleeding disorders or anticoagulant therapy. To prevent skin necrosis the ring should be removed soon after intercourse.

INTRA-CAVERNOSAL INJECTIONS (2ND LINE)

Alprostadil can be delivered as injection into corpora cavernosa – patient must be suitably trained.

Caverject / Viridal are available preparations.

Should be given as mono-therapy in doses of 5–40μg.

Efficacy rates > 70% are reported.

Most common side effect is penile pain which is self-limiting, other include priapism and fibrosis, and the development of Peyronie's should indicate stopping therapy indefinitely.

Most drop-outs occur within 3 months of commencing treatment.

INTRA-URETHRAL ALPROSTADIL (MUSE) (2ND LINE)

Alprostadil is a synthetic prostaglandin.

Can be provided as 500μg – 1000μg doses to be used on demand.

Efficacy lower than intra-cavernosal treatment (<65%), however may be preferable as less invasive, and can be augmented by use of constricting ring at penile base.

Local pain is the most common side effect.

TOPICAL ALPROSTADIL (2ND LINE)

Similar preparation of alprostadil that can be delivered as a cream into urethra – dosage of 300μ.

SHOCKWAVE LITHOTRIPSY

ESWL has been recommended to treat ED, on premise that it may promote neo-vascularisation.

EAU Guidelines do not provide clear recommendations with regard to its use.

PENILE PROSTHESES (3RD LINE)

Surgical implantation of a penile prosthesis should be considered in patients:
- fail / unwilling / unable to consider 1st and 2nd line treatment options

- severe Peyronie's disease
- penile fibrosis (eg. after priapism)
- penile trauma

The available options are malleable or inflatable devices.

Malleable devices can be manually placed into erect or flaccid state.

Inflatable devices often preferred as they allow more "natural" erections to be obtained.

3-piece inflatable device consists of reservoir placed in retro-pubic space (auto-inflation is less likely) and filled with saline, pump placed in scrotum and pair of cylinders within the corpora of penis.

Satisfaction rates with penile prosthesis, regardless of the cause, are ≥ 90%.

The *side-effects* of penile prosthesis surgery include:
- infection, erosion, mechanical failure (< 5%)
- glans droop (may require glanspexy)

Infection rate (< 5%) most commonly due to staphyloccal organisms, higher in diabetic patients and those taking steroid medication (≤ 50%)

Severe infection will require that the implant needs removing – delayed re-insertion may be more challenging due to fibrosis.

The *Mulcahy technique* is a 7-step strategy washout system involving a series of anti-microbial agents and mechanical lavage of all spaces (reservoir space, corpora). [11]

ED POST RADICAL PROSTATECTOMY

The use of pro-erectile drugs after RP is important in achieving post-operative erectile function.

Higher rates of erectile function recovery after RP have been shown in patients receiving any drug (therapeutic or prophylactic) for ED (penile rehabilitation).

PDE5i are considered 1st line after RP – although such patients are considered poor-responders.

More invasive options are intra-cavernosal injections (2nd line) and prosthesis (3rd line).

HYPOGONADISM

Hypogonadism in itself can be:

- *primary*, due to testicular failure (e.g. mumps orchitis, chemo/radio therapy, trauma)
- *secondary*, due to insufficient GnRH / FSH / LH (e.g. Kallman's syndrome, pituitary pathology)
- androgen insensitivity

Late-onset hypogonadism (LOH) is defined as a clinical and biochemical syndrome associated with advancing age and characterised by symptoms of testosterone deficiency.

PATHOPHYSIOLOGY

Ageing decreases the production of LHRH and LH.

This causes a decline in both number of Leydig cells and their sensitivity to LH.

DIAGNOSTIC EVALUATION

PATIENT HISTORY

The following symptoms are common in LOH:
- ED, reduced libido
- lethargy, poor concentration, change in mood, sleep disturbance
- loss of muscle mass, osteoporosis
- hair loss, skin changes

PATIENT EXAMINATION

This should be thorough and performed in the presence of a chaperone.

The following aspects should be assessed:
- general examination to assess posture, BMI and hair distribution
- presence of gynaecomastia
- DRE
- soft and small volume testes

Testicular volume > 16mL (average ~ 20mL):

- Interstitial tissue ~ 20–30% of total (Leydig cells, blood vessels, lymphatics)
- Germ cell lines constitute the remainder

BASELINE INVESTIGATIONS

Blood tests should be performed to include LH / FSH, testosterone (8am and 11am are preferred as levels peak) and prolactin.

Include fasting glucose and lipid profile.

A DEXA scan can be considered to assess for bone mineral density (osteoporosis).

SHBG

If testosterone is low, consider measuring the SHBG.

SHBG naturally binds approximately 45% of total circulating testosterone in healthy young men, which is tightly bound and not available for tissue use.

Bio-available testosterone = (free testosterone ~ 2%) + (albumin-bound testosterone)

SHBG can increase with age (reflecting the natural fall in free testosterone).

SHBG can be affected by cirrhosis, hyperthyroidism, oestrogen use and HIV.

Testosterone half-life is ~ 15 minutes, metabolised by the liver and conjugated to glucuronides which are excreted renally.

MANAGEMENT

Hypogonadism with related symptoms should be treated with testosterone replacement therapy (TRT) as long as no contra-indications.

Contra-indications to TRT include:

- active prostate or breast cancer
- primary liver tumour
- clinically significant BPH (LUTS may worsen)
- polycythaemia (TRT can further increase haematocrit)
- severe liver / renal / heart failure (testosterone increases water and potassium retention)

Prior to commencing TRT therefore you should perform:
- DRE and PSA
- lipid profile
- LFT, UEs, haematocrit
- consider DEXA scan (for comparison)

As the treatment progresses you should perform annual DRE, PSA, FBC. [12]

The most common abnormality is raised haematocrit which will settle if TRT stopped (the highest risk of this is noted with IM administration).

Methods available for delivering TRT are categorised in [Table 7].

TRT should not be used to treat infertility in the context of hypogonadism.

After cessation of TRT, the symptoms related to its deficiency are likely to return.

Table 7 – Comparison of different administration routes for TRT

Route	Dose
Oral	120mg daily dose
Intra-muscular	1000mg at 6 and 12 weeks, 1000mg every 3 months
Trans-dermal	Daily gel or patch (5–10mg)
Sub-dermal	T-pellets (200mg every 5 months)

LUTS DIAGNOSTIC EVALUATION

PATIENT HISTORY

A complete medical history must be taken from men with LUTS.

All published guidelines for male LUTS / BPH recommend using validated symptom score questionnaire to quantify LUTS and identify predominant symptoms.

International Prostate Symptom Score (IPSS) features:

- 7 symptom questions
- 1 quality of life (QOL) question
- score is asymptomatic (0), "mild" (1–7), "moderate" (8–19) and "severe" (20–35)
- allows for re-evaluation during / after treatment

An increase > 4 points on the IPSS is related to a subjective worsening of bother of urinary symptoms.

Alternatives include the Danish Prostate Symptom Score and AUA Symptom Score.

STATION 8: BPH AND ANDROLOGY

Table 8 – IPSS questionnaire and additional quality of life question

In the past month:	Not at all	Less than 1/5 times	Less than ½ the time	About ½ the time	More than ½ the time	Almost always
1. Incomplete emptying How often have you had a sensation of not emptying your bladder completely after you finish urinating?	0	1	2	3	4	5
2. Frequency How often have you had to urinate again less than two hours after you finished urinating?	0	1	2	3	4	5
3. Intermittency How often have you found you stopped and started again several times when you urinated?	0	1	2	3	4	5
4. Urgency How difficult have you found it to postpone going to pass urine?	0	1	2	3	4	5
5. Weak stream How often have you had a weak urinary stream?	0	1	2	3	4	5
6. Straining How often have you had to push or strain to begin urination?	0	1	2	3	4	5
	None	Once	Twice	3 x	4 x	≥ 5 x
7. Nocturia How many times did you most typically get up to urinate from bedtime until waking up in morning?	0	1	2	3	4	5

Quality of life question	Delighted	Pleased	Mostly satisfied	Mixed	Mostly dissatisfied	Unhappy	Terrible
If you were to live the rest of your life with your urinary symptoms as they are now, how would you feel?	0	1	2	3	4	5	6

PATIENT EXAMINATION

A thorough examination should be undertaken in the presence of a chaperone.

Ensure that examination assess for:

- general, signs of renal failure (fluid overload) or neurological disease (gait, tremors)
- abdominal, for palpable bladder, ballotable kidneys, scars
- DRE, size / consistency / tenderness of the prostate

BASELINE INVESTIGATIONS

The recommended tests will depend on the history of condition and red-flag symptoms.

For a moderate LUTS severity in the absence of red-flag symptoms, consider:

1. Urinanalysis and MSU for culture as appropriate
2. Frequency-Volume Chart / Bladder diary – for 3 days
3. Uroflowmetry and PVR measurement

PSA testing should not be offered routinely (unless abnormal DRE, positive family history, patient request) and the patient counselled appropriately.

Serum creatinine and eGFR warranted if suspected renal impairment (eg. stones, recurrent UTIs)

Routine renal US should not be performed unless:

- recurrent UTI / sterile pyuria

- haematuria
- profound symptoms or pain
- chronic retention

Routine flexible cystoscopy should not be performed unless:
- rUTI / sterile pyuria
- haematuria
- profound symptoms or pain

Routine TRUS evaluation of the prostate should not be performed unless:
- abnormal DRE or PSA

Routine UDS should not be performed unless:
- previous failed invasive LUTS treatment / surgery
- co-existing neurological disease
- men who cannot void > 150mL
- considering surgery in men with predominantly voiding LUTS and PVR > 300mL
- considering surgery in men with predominantly voiding LUTS and age > 80y or < 50y

Recall the relevant ICS nomogram based on UDS findings as per Figure 3 below.

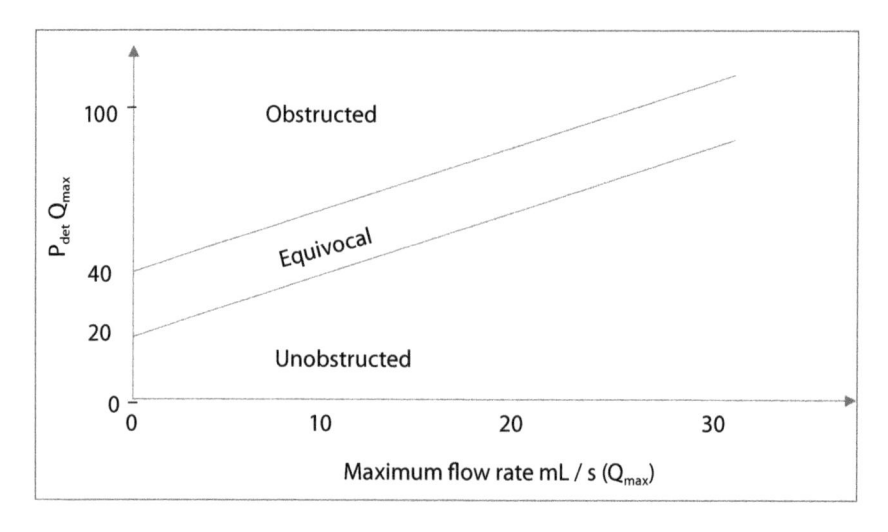

Figure 3 – ICS nomogram based on UDS findings

Bladder Outlet Obstruction Index (Abrams-Grifiths number) = $P_{det}Q_{max} - 2Q_{max}$
- obstructed < 20, equivocal 20–40, obstructed > 40

UROFLOWMETRY

This can be affected by age, race and voided volume (ideally > 150mL and < 500mL).

Normal age-specific flow rates (Q_{max}) for men:
- < 40 years = > 21mL / s
- 40 60 years = > 18mL / s
- > 60 years = > 13mL / s

Normal age-specific flow rates (Q_{max}) for women:
- < 50 years = > 25mL / s
- > 50 years = < 18mL / s

A reduced Q_{max} is usually evidence of BOO.

90% of men with Q_{max} < 10mL / s will have urodynamic evidence of obstruction, the remaining 10% will have evidence of reduced detrusor contractility.

75% of men with Q_{max} > 15mL / s will not have BOO (the remaining 25% who are obstructed maintain their flow by having increased detrusor work).

As an approximate guide to uroflowmetry interpretation:
- Q_{max} < 10mL / s   = 90% chance of obstruction
- Q_{max} 10–15mL / s   = 60% chance of obstruction
- Q_{max} > 15mL / s   = 10% chance of obstruction

EPIDEMIOLOGY

Prevalence of BPH varies according to definition used.

Studies which define BPH on symptoms alone give higher prevalence than those which necessitate a Q_{max} reduction or objective prostatic enlargement.

The *Olmsted County study* showed prevalence of moderate / severe LUTS in 28% > 70 years.

UK estimated that > 20g prostate with symptoms or reduced Q_{max} in 43% aged 60–69 years.

INFERTILITY

MALE REPRODUCTIVE PHYSIOLOGY

The hypothalamic-pituitary-gonadal axis is shown in diagram below.

GnRH (or LHRH) from hypothalamus causes pulsatile release of FSH / LH from anterior pituitary which in turn acts on the testis.

LH makes Leydig cells produce testosterone, FSH stimulates inhibin and sperm production.

In blood, testosterone is free (2%), bound to albumin (38%) and bound to SHBG (60%).

In androgen-responsive tissues, 5 α-reductase converts testosterone to its more potent form DHT.

Testosterone provides the primary negative feedback hormone to pituitary LH.

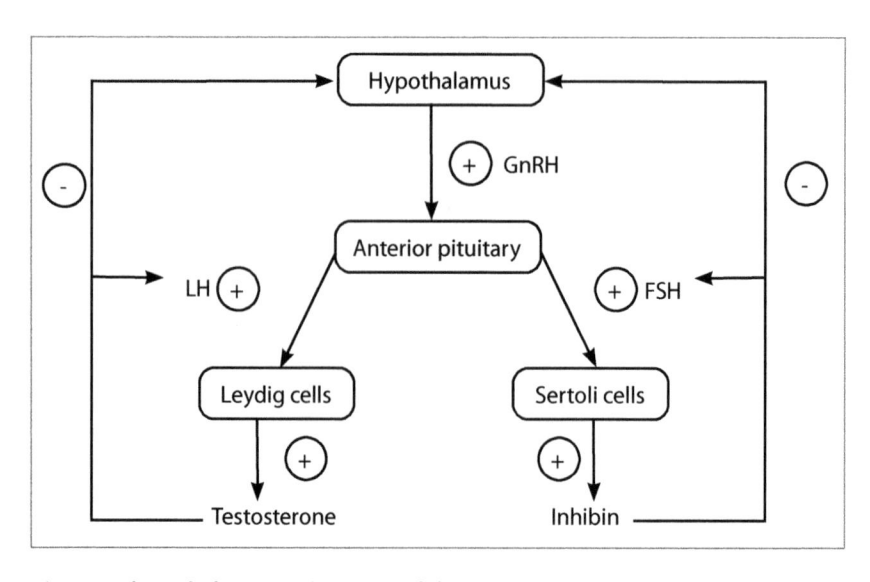

Figure 4 – hypothalamo-pituitary gonadal axis

SPERMATOGENESIS

Seminiferous tubules are lined with Sertoli cells, which provide nutrients to germ cells.

Type-A spermatogonia are stem cells – they can self-renew (remaining as type-A) or differentiate to sperm (type-B).

Primordial germ cells

(x1 type-B spermatogonium) → mitosis → primary spermatocytes (x2 diploid)

(1st meiotic division) → secondary spermatocytes (46 chromosomes) (x4)

(2nd meiotic division) → spermatids (23 chromosomes) (x8)

(spermiogenesis) → spermatozoa (entire process 72 days)

i.e. one type-B spermatogonium will yield 8 spermatozoa

These are stored and matured in the epididymis, however they spend most of their life in the testis.

Sperm motility increases during epididymal transit, due to increased capacity for glycolysis.

Sperm is viable for ≤ 5 days in the female.

DEFINITIONS

Infertility defined as inability to achieve pregnancy within 12 months of regular unprotected sex

Azoospermia, absent sperm in ejaculate

Oligospermia, abnormality of low sperm numbers (< 15 x 10^6 / mL)

Asthenospermia, abnormality of motility (< 40% motile), progressive motility < 32%

Teratozoospermia, abnormality of morphology (< 4% normal forms)

Globozoospermia, sperm lack acrosomal caps (rendered spherical), natural conception is not possible and would require ICSI

Necrospermia, high percentage of dead / immotile sperm (test with vitality staining)

OAT syndrome, refers to combined defects of sperm motility, morphology and density (oligoasthenoteratospermia) can be caused by varicocoele, cryptorchidism, heat.

EPIDEMIOLOGY

Chance of normal couple conceiving is 20% / month (90% in one year).

Infertility is caused by male factors alone (20%), female factors alone (50%) and both female and male factors (30%).

Azoospermia is present in 1% of male population.

SEMEN CHARACTERISTICS

Accurate semen analysis is an important test for evaluation of the infertile male.

Recommended that patient abstains from ejaculation for 2–5 days prior to sample.

Sample should be provided in clean container (ideally directly in laboratory), or with delay ≤ 1 hour to delivery of sample (kept warm in transit), without use of condoms (spermicide).

Any repeat sample should be delivered ≥ 3 months from last (full spermatogenesis cycle).

Coitus interruptus sample not recommended as acidic vaginal secretions may contaminate this.

The majority of the ejaculate volume is derived from the seminal vesicles (~70%).

The WHO (2010) defined the reference values for various different facets of a semen analysis. [Table 9]

Table 9 – WHO (2010) semen analysis parameters [14]

Parameter	Lower reference limit (range)
Semen volume (mL)	> 1.5
Total sperm count (10^6)	> 39
Sperm concentration (10^6/ mL)	> 15
Progressive motility (PR %)	> 32
Vitality (live spermatozoa %)	> 58
Sperm morphology (normal forms, %)	> 4
pH	> 7.2

The *mixed agglutination reaction* (MAR) test is used to detect anti-sperm antibodies, which can be useful in immunological infertility.

Distribution of male infertility by semen analysis:
- Multiple abnormalities 49%
- Normal 14%
- Azoospermia 14%
- Single abnormality: Low vol. 7% Asthenospermia 6% Teratospermia 4% Oligospermia 4%

Further evaluation of male infertility should be directed towards the predominant semen finding.

AETIOLOGY

There are many causes of male factor infertility.
- *Idiopathic,* seen in ≤ 25% of cases
- *congenital,* such as anorchia, cryptorchidism, genetic (eg. Klinefelter, Kartagener, CF)
- *trauma*
- *testicular torsion*
- *hormonal,* such as prolactinoma, steroid abuse, CAH, low FSH / LH / testosterone
- *systemic,* such as liver / renal failure
- *varicocoele*
- *previous chemotherapy*
- *infective,* such as STIs, mumps orchitis (no association with HIV and adverse sperm function)
- recreational drugs, such as anabolic steroids and marijuana

The top 3 male factors: varicocoele, idiopathic and obstructive (endocrine only accounts for ~ 2%).

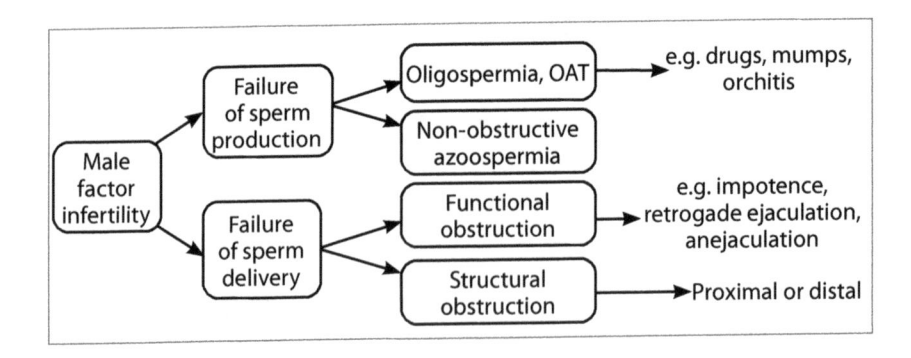

Figure 5 – male factor infertility

DIAGNOSTIC EVALUATION

PATIENT HISTORY

The history must be thorough and consider the partner of the patient, ideally in a dedicated fertility clinic with a fertility nurse specialist present:

- duration of infertility and frequency of intercourse
- details of previous conceptions / births
- timing of coitus
- erectile and ejaculatory function
- use of vaginal lubricants (can be spermicidal)
- sexual development history

The detailed past medical and drug history should screen for risk factors as listed above.

PATIENT EXAMINATION

The patient must be examined thoroughly in the presence of a chaperone.

Commence by general inspection – assessing for BMI, signs of development of secondary sexual characteristics / virilisation pattern.

After this a focused urological examination should be performed:

- testes, are these palpable, bilateral and normal in size
- presence of varicocoele
- vas deferens, are these both palpable in the scrotum
- epididymis, signs of blockage / granuloma

INFERTILITY

The partner should undergo full assessment in a dedicated gynaecological clinic for infertility.

A longitudinal axis < 4.6cm measured with caliper orchidometer is associated with potential impairment in spermatogenesis.

INVESTIGATIONS

BASELINE

The following blood tests should be performed: LH, FSH and testosterone (as well as viral screen e.g. hepatitis B and C, HIV).

Interpretation of their results are shown in [Table 10].

Table 10 – Diagnostic interpretation of combined FSH, LH and testosterone results

FSH	LH	Testosterone	Diagnosis
High	Normal	Nomal	Seminiferous tubule damage
Normal	Normal	Normal	Genital tract obstruction
High	High	Normal	Testicular failure
Low	Low	Low	Hypogonadotrophism

i.e. raised FSH suggests testes not working, reduced FSH suggests intra-cranial pathology, normal FSH value could suggest obstructive cause.

Two separate semen analyses are recommended to confirm an abnormal result. Compare values to those standardised in WHO parameters (table above).

Ensure at least 3 days of abstinence prior to semen sample delivery.

Pasqualini syndrome – isolated deficiency in LH

IMAGING

Scrotal US may evaluate testicular abnormalities and detection of varicocoele.

Trans-rectal US is indicated in low ejaculate volumes to investigate obstruction of seminal vesicles or ejaculatory ducts.

VASOGRAPHY

A vasogram involves puncture of vas deferens within scrotum and injection of contrast, which if normal should flow freely through vas into bladder.

Should be done ideally at time of planned reconstructive surgery (vas damage may occur that might complicate future surgery).

TESTICULAR BIOPSY

Performed in azoospermia to differentiate between obstructive and non-obstructive causes

Sperm can be retrieved simultaneously for use in assisted conception (AC), as long as it is sufficiently mature on the *Johnsen score* (≥ 8, range 1–10).

Biopsy is rarely performed in isolation.

Biopsy is not routinely indicated in oligospermia as it does not affect treatment options.

Biopsy is not routinely indicated in azoospermia if normal testes volume and gonadotrophins and CBAVD – patient needs counselling for cystic fibrosis screening followed by TESE.

The Johnsen score count is used to classify spermatogenesis on a testicular biopsy [Table 11]

Table 11 – Johnsen score used as histological grading system for testicular biopsy

Score	Description
1	No cells, tubular fibrosis
2	Sertoli cells only
3	Spermatogonia
4	< 10 spermatocytes
5	No spermatozoa, many spermatocytes
6	No spermatozoa, but < 10 spermatids
7	No spermatozoa, but many spermatids
8	< 10 spermatozoa
9	Many spermatozoa – disorganised epithelium
10	Complete spermatogenesis

OLIGOSPERMIA

Defined as sperm concentration $< 15 \times 10^6$ / mL of ejaculate

- If < 10, consider karyotyping
- If < 5, consider Y-microdeletion test

Common causes include varicocoele, androgen deficiency and idiopathic.

Along with the history taken in context, the following tests should be considered:

- hormone profile (raised FSH may suggest seminiferous tubular failure)
- serum prolactin (hyper-prolactinaemia may adversely affect spermatogenesis)
- US scrotum to evaluate for varicocoele

Isolated FSH elevation indicates failure of spermatogenesis rather than endocrine abnormality.

Treatment mainly involves addressing underlying cause (if found) or AC.

AZOOSPERMIA

Defined as absence of sperm within the ejaculate, can be obstructive (40%) vs. non-obstructive (60%)

The following are obstructive causes:

- vas deferens, such as CBAVD (associated with renal agenesis and cystic fibrosis), vasectomy, previous scrotal / hernia surgery
- epididymal, such as post-infective or post-surgery
- ejaculatory duct (e.g. anejaculation in spinal cord injury)

Obstructive causes are more common in patients with normal testes and hormone profile, with a semen analysis suggesting azoospermia.

The following are non-obstructive causes:

- hormonal, such as hypogonadotrophism
- abnormalities of spermatogenesis, such as trauma / torsion, mumps, Klinefelter's

INVESTIGATIONS

Hormone profile blood tests (LH / FSH / testosterone) which should all return normal

Semen samples (x 2) to confirm diagnosis

Trans-rectal US can assess vas and /or ejaculatory duct obstruction

Vasogram and testicular biopsy as discussed previously

Chromosomal analyses are not routinely recommended, consider if Klinefelter's is suspected (azoospermia, small testes, low FSH /LH / testosterone, gynaecomastia).

Table 12 – Test result profile for different aetiological causes of azoospermia

	Distal obstruction	Proximal obstruction	Retrograde Ejaculation	Anejaculation (e.g. spinal cord injury
FSH	normal	normal	normal	normal
Testes volume	normal	normal	normal	normal
Semen volume	normal	Low	low / none	none
Sperm count	azoospermia	azoospermia	azoospermia	azoospermia
Fructose / pH	normal	low, acidic	normal	n/a
Post-ejaculate urinanalysis	normal	Normal	> 10 sperm / HPF	n/a

MANAGEMENT

The management plan will depend on the underlying cause that has been identified.

CBAVD will require AC techniques.

If a tubular obstructive cause is identified, then surgical excision and anastomosis can be performed (microsurgical vaso-vasostomy or tubulo-vasostomy).

Ejaculatory Duct Obstruction

Uncommon, accounting for < 5% of male infertility cases due to obstructive causes

May arise congenitally (Mullerian or Wolffian duct cysts) or acquired (calculus)

Findings may include azoo / oligo- spermia with low semen fructose / volume / pH; TRUS evaluation may reveal dilated seminal vesicles

Ejaculatory duct obstruction is treated by *trans-urethral resection of ejaculatory ducts* (TURED).

The seminal vesicals are filled with methylene blue (via trans-rectal needle), the surgeon then resects the verumontanum until a blue flush is seen.

Patency rates ≤ 90%, fertility ≤ 40%

Y MICRO-DELETION

In the context of male infertility, Y-chromosome micro-deletions are usually phenotypically normal, with the only abnormality being a defect in spermatogenesis.

The defect occurs in one of three non-overlapping regions of the long arm of Y-chromosome.

These are referred to as AZFa (proximal), AZFb (middle) and AZFc (distal).

The following are associated:

- AZFa micro-deletion – Sertoli only (cannot father children)
- AZFb micro-deletion – maturation arrest (cannot father children)
- AZFc micro-deletion – severe oligospermia (50% success rate with micro-TESE, however all male offspring will be infertile)

Men with AZF a or b will not have sperm within testicle and therefore retrieval is not indicated, whilst there is a small chance (10%) of finding sperm in AZFc.

All male offspring of men with micro-deletions will inherit the same deletion.

AZFa/b have to be advised regarding sperm donation or adoption.

MALE ASSISTED CONCEPTION

There are many AC techniques as listed in [Table 12].

Table 13 – Techniques of AC and their abbreviations

Technique	Abbreviation
Intra-uterine insemination	IUI
In-vitro fertilisation	IVF
Intra-cytoplasmic sperm injection	ICSI
Microsurgical epididymal sperm aspiration	MESA
Percutaneous sperm aspiration	PESA
Testicular sperm extraction	TESE
Micro testicular sperm extraction	mTESE
Testicular sperm aspiration	TESA

INTRAUTERINE INSEMINATION (IUI)

Used to bypass cervical mucus (sperm placed directly into uterus)

Sperm must be processed to remove prostaglandins (very irritant to uterus) and bacteria, often with ovarian hyper-stimulation to improve pregnancy rate.

Indications:
- Deposition abnormality (hypospadias) Cervical factor
- Severe dyspareunia
- Severe psychosexual abnormality

Requirements:
- 5–10 million/mL motile sperm (up to 50% loss after processing)

Outcome:
- Pregnancy rates of up to 30% for 4 cycles
- Multiple gestation in up to 30%

IVF AND ICSI

Ovarian hyper-stimulation with clomiphene and trans-vaginal egg harvest

Petri dish fertilisation, 2–3 day growth, followed by trans-cervical blastocyst implantation. One third of implanted embryos survive

IVF less than 5 million/mL sperm, which are mixed with retrieved oocytes and incubated for 2–3 days prior to trans-cervical placement into uterus

ICSI one sperm required injected directly into the oocyte cytoplasm through zone pellicida

Outcome

Pregnancy rate 20–30% per cycle, significantly related to age

SPERM RETRIEVAL TECHNIQUES

Sperm retrieval techniques are indicated when reconstruction is not possible.

MESA or PESA – equivalent pregnancy rates

MESA is more invasive but retrieves more sperm, therefore can be frozen.

No difference in pregnancy rates after ICSI with fresh vs. frozen

TESE conventionally involves single / multiple testicular biopsies to retrieve seminiferous tubules, which are then dissected to retrieve mature sperm to use for AC.

mTESE utilises high magnification of seminiferous tubules to target the best ones for extraction, which can then be frozen for future ICSI or sperm harvested for same day ICSI cycle.

PEYRONIE'S DISEASE

Peyronie's disease (PD) is an acquired condition characterised by deformity of the penile shaft secondary to the formation of a fibrous scar on the tunica albuginea.

EPIDEMIOLOGY

Congenital penile curvature is rare (< 1%) – any correction should be deferred until after puberty.

PD is likely under-reported – estimated prevalence ≤ 10%.

Definite PD prevalent ≤ 1% (higher prevalence amongst diabetics)

Typical age of patient with PD 50–60 years.

48% of patients with PD have mild / moderate depression, 25% have Dupuytren's contracture.

AETIOLOGY

Exact cause unknown

Considered to be a wound-healing disorder which occurs after penile trauma in predisposed men, due to micro-vascular injury / bleeding into tunica resulting in inflammation and fibrosis

Natural progression of PD:
- 40% progress within 1 year,
- 14% resolve spontaneously,
- 50% approximately experience stabilisation

The plaques have extensive connective tissue with random collagen orientation (most common dorsally) – *transforming growth factor beta* (TGF-β1) is over-expressed.

Two phases of the disease can be distinguished: *Active / inflammatory* and *Stable / fibrotic*.

Often occurs in concomitance with ED, due to altered haemodynamics of cavernosal blood flow

Active Phase

The acute inflammatory phase will last ≤ 6 months.

Patient may experience pain in flaccid and / or erect state, the curvature will start to develop along with palpable plaque.

Stable Phase

The chronic fibrotic phase lasts subsequently ≤ 12 months.

The pain disappears for most (90%) and the curvature should stop progressing further, spontaneous improvement is unusual (14%).

Treatment should be deferred until the stable phase is established.

RISK FACTORS

The most commonly associated co-morbidities with PD are:
- diabetes
- smoking and excessive alcohol
- hypertension, IHD, lipid abnormalities
- Dupuytren's contracture (present in 25% of PD patients)
- Ledderhose's disease (plantar-fascial contracture)
- previous penile trauma

DIAGNOSTIC EVALUATION

PATIENT HISTORY

The patient history and examination are key to diagnosing PD.

Key factors to be established in the history include:
- duration and progression of symptoms
- presence of pain (active vs. stable disease)
- evidence of erectile dysfunction
- degree of curvatures (photographic evidence may be available)
- risk factors and associated co-morbidities

Ask patient to complete validated questionnaire such as IIEF-5 (although this has not been formally validated for Peyronie's disease).

There is an alternative "Peyronie's disease questionnaire". [14]

PATIENT EXAMINATION

The examination of the patient should be conducted in the presence of a chaperone.

Examination of external genitalia should be performed for palpable plaque (more common on dorsal aspect) whose size does not correlate with degree of curvature.

Examine hands and feet for evidence of Dupuytren's contracture or Ledderhose scarring.

An objective assessment of penile curvature with an erection is mandatory:
- degree of curvature
- measurement of flaccid and erect penile length (important if surgery is planned)

US not recommended to measure plaque, Doppler may only be relevant for vascular parameters.

Medical photography with signed consent is preferable: lateral, frontal and views from above.

MANAGEMENT

CONSERVATIVE

Non-operative management is advocated for early PD (during active phase).

PD in itself does not mandate treatment if patient is not troubled by condition, common symptoms that impact QOL include ED and inability to penetrate.

A small proportion of cases (14%) will resolve spontaneously, and half will not progress.

MEDICAL

There are many proposed medical options available to treat PD, however most have not undergone rigorous evaluation in controlled clinical trials.

Most agents rely on anecdotal evidence to support their usage.

ESWL

Possibly works by damaging / remodelling the plaque, or by increasing the vascularity.

May help to reduce pain however not beneficial for curvature.

NICE Guidelines do not recommend unless patient counselled regarding low success rate.

Tamoxifen

Oestrogen receptor antagonist that modulates TGFβ-1 secretion by fibroblasts, believed to be more effective in the acute inflammatory phase

EAU Guidelines do not recommend.

Intra-lesional Treatment

Injecting steroids into the lesion are thought to oppose the inflammatory process and decrease collagen synthesis at the cost of tissue thinning.

EAU Guidelines do not recommend.

POTABA

Drug used to treat disorders associated with formation of excess fibrous tissue in the body (e.g. Peyronie's, scleroderma)

Works by increasing the uptake of oxygen into the tissue [15]

Administered as potassium para-aminobenzoate – 3g (PO) QDS

Vitamin-E

Works by inactivating free radicals that saturate NO, thereby keeping active NO levels elevated to promote wound healing and offer anti-inflammatory action by limiting oxidative stress [16]

Given as 200mg TDS for 3 months

May improve pain in ≤ 75% and deformity in ≤ 12 %

Clostridium Collagenase (CCH)

CCH (marketed as Xiapex™) as injection is the only drug approved for the treatment of PD by the FDA and NICE.

CCH is an enzyme that attacks collagen (primary component of PD plaque).

CCH injection may cause penile pain, bruising and swelling as most common side effects.

Different regimens of prescribing available, number of injections will vary, there will be period of penile modelling in between injections to complete one cycle of treatment (may require multiple cycles)

Penile Traction Devices

Traction and / or vacuum devices have been shown to beneficial in the pre- and post- operative PD setting, alone or in conjunction with other treatments.

Can increase / preserve penile length, encourages tissue modelling, must be used ≥ 3 hours / day

SURGICAL

Surgery is indicated in patients with stable PD (≥ 3 months) and erections where the condition does not allow for satisfactory sexual intercourse.

Assessment of erectile function (IIEF-5 score), flaccid / erect penile length and angle of curvature (photo record) are important considerations in patient work-up.

Choice of procedure between convex shortening (Nesbit / Yachia / plication) or concave lengthening (plaque incision and grafting) with or without prosthesis insertion for ED

Penile (Convex) Shortening Surgery

Penile shortening procedures involve plication techniques (e.g. Nesbit) also called corporoplasty.

Plication surgery is generally recommended in mild / moderate PD (< 60°) with good erections.

Nesbit procedure involves:
- de-gloving of penis via circumglanular incision
- induction of artificial erection to reveal site of maximal deformity
- opposite side excise tissue ellipse (1mm for every 10° curve), close defect with sutures

All patients will experience penile shortening.

Success rates > 80%, recurrence uncommon and ED rare (1%)

Yachia procedure is a less common alternative – involves multiple longitudinal incisions in tunica which are closed horizontally.

Penile (Concave) Lengthening Surgery

Penile lengthening procedures involve excision / incision of plaque with defect filled by a graft.

Incision undertaken in the short (concave) side to increase this side's length, with the aim of relaxing the tunica completely

Lue procedure involves plaque incision with insertion of venous patch to lengthen affected side:

- saphenous vein is the most common autograft (followed by dorsal penile vein)
- alternative graft materials include auto- (tunica vaginalis), allo- (cadaveric pericardium), xeno- grafts (porcine small intestine) or synthetic

Lue procedure has higher risk of ED (15%), much lower of penile shortening ($\leq$ 20%).

Penile Implants

Penile implants are an option for severe PD. [see ED notes]

Inflatable prostheses are generally preferred by patients over malleable, good long-term satisfaction rates 79–100% with inflatables.

The risk of urethral injury (5%) is much greater during prosthesis insertion in PD than non-PD.

Deformities $\leq$ 30° after implant insertion are likely to resolve once pump is used for 6 months.

Severe hourglass deformity with good erectile function, may require grafting and penile prosthesis

PD SURGERY ALGORITHM

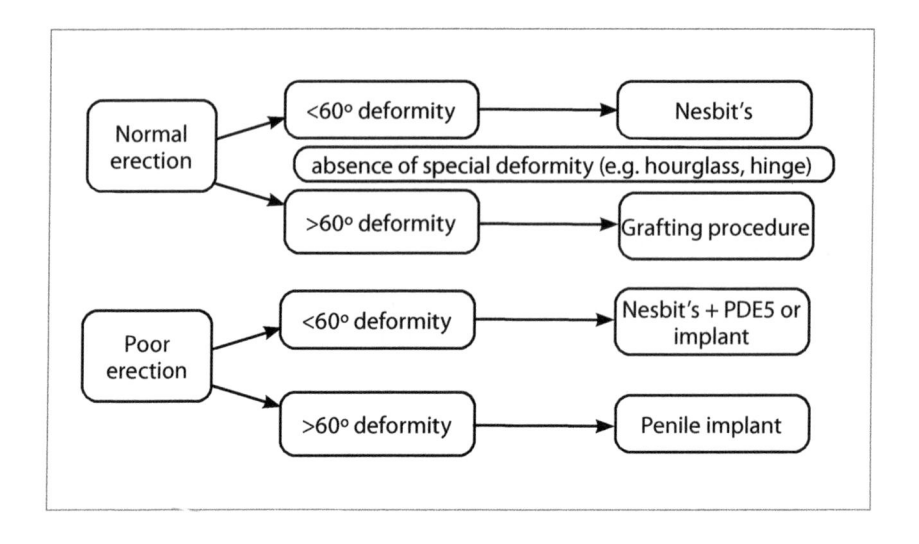

- Normal erection
  - <60° deformity → Nesbit's
  - absence of special deformity (e.g. hourglass, hinge)
  - >60° deformity → Grafting procedure
- Poor erection
  - <60° deformity → Nesbit's + PDE5 or implant
  - >60° deformity → Penile implant

Figure 6 – PD surgery algorithm

TREATMENT OF BPH

WATCHFUL WAITING

Many men with LUTS are not sufficiently troubled by their symptoms to need treatment.

Watchful waiting (WW) is a viable option for such men, as few progress to urinary retention and related complications, even if their IPSS score is severe.

Symptoms are likely to deteriorate with age, however the overall extent of this is low.

The QOL impact score is most relevant – only treat if symptoms are bothering the patient.

PSA is a helpful independent marker for predicting disease progression in BPH, if ≥ 1.4ng / mL indicates increased risk of disease progression.

Other factors that can predict disease progression include:
- failure to respond to medical therapy
- symptom deterioration whilst on treatment
- increasing PVR
- presence of inflammation on TRUS biopsies

Counsel patient about lifestyle measures, such as fluid intake advice.

MEDICAL THERAPY

α-1 ADRENORECEPTOR ANTAGONISTS

Inhibit effect of noradrenaline on smooth muscle in the prostate by blocking α-1 adrenoreceptors (α-1 AR) thereby reducing tone

α-1 blockers have little effect of urodynamically determined BOO.

There are 2 broad sub-types of α-adrenoreceptor (α-1 and α-2), and 3 sub-types of α-1 AR (α1-a, α-1b and α1L).

The α-1 blockers are classified by their AR selectivity and elimination half-life. [Table 14]

Table 14 – the different classifications of α-1 blockers

Selectivity	α-1 blocker
Non-selective	Phenoxybenzamine
α-1	Prazosin, alfuzosin
Long acting α-1	terazosin, doxazosin
Sub-type selective α-1a (more than α-1b)	Tamsulosin

All α-1 blockers have similar efficacy in appropriate doses.

Efficacy

Benefits can be noted within hours / days, full effect takes several weeks.

If a ≥ 25% reduction in IPSS is considered successful, response rates of 30–40% can be seen with α-1 blockers.

This equates to 4–5 points improvement in score over placebo.

Side-Effects

The most common side-effects of α-1 blockers include:

- asthenia (weakness)
- dizziness and postural hypotension
- retrograde ejaculation
- floppy iris syndrome during cataract surgery (i.e. inform ophthalmologist), risk may not disappear even if medication is stopped

5α-REDUCTASE INHIBITORS

5α-RI work on the static component of BPE, achieving prostatic volume reduction over months.

Testosterone is converted to DHT which has more potent androgenic effects on the prostate, this process is mediated by the enzyme 5α-reductase.

There are 2 isoforms of the 5α-reductase enzyme:

- *type-1*, minor expression in prostate (mainly in skin and liver)
- *type-2*, predominant expression and activity in the prostate

5α-RI work by competitive inhibition of the enzyme to reduce testosterone conversion to DHT.

Two 5α-RI are available for clinical use – dutasteride (type 1 and 2) and finasteride (type 2 only).

- serum reduction of DHT with dutasteride (95%) and finasteride (70%)
- prostate DHT reduction similar for both around 90%

EAU Guidelines recommend 5α-RI for patients with moderate / severe LUTS and prostate > 40mL

Patients must be counselled regarding the delayed symptomatic improvement with 5α-RI.

Finasteride are less effective when used as mono-therapy when compared to α-1 blockers, however they help reduce disease progression.

PLESS Study: 55% reduction in need for TURP, 57% reduced AUR incidence over 4 years

- (NNT = 25 of finasteride to prevent AUR) [17]

Efficacy

5α-RI (not α-1 blockers) reduce long-term risk of AUR (57%) or outflow surgery (55%) at 4 years.

After 2–4 years of 5α-RI treatment:

- IPSS improvement of 15–30%
- decrease prostate volume ≤ 28%
- increase Q_{max} by ≤ 2mL / s

Finasteride is comparable to placebo for prostates < 40mL (however mild benefit for dutasteride).

5α-RI may reduce bleeding during TURP surgery due to effects on prostatic re-vascularisation (suppression of VEGF).

Side-Effects

Generally mild and related to sexual function

Erectile dysfunction, reduced libido, gynaecomastia (1–2%) and ejaculation disorders

Recall the findings from the PCPT trial, where lower prevalance of PCa in finasteride group noted (however higher incidence of high-grade tumours)

COMBINATION THERAPY

Combination therapies refer to 5α-RI plus α-1 blocker.

BAUS Guidelines suggest combination therapy for men with:
- bothersome LUTS
- prostatic obstruction
- risk factors for disease progression (enlarged prostate > 30mL, Q_{max} < 12mL/s, increasing PVR and PSA)

Several trials have evaluated efficacy of combination therapy.

MTOPS (Medical Therapy Of Prostatic Symptoms)

Double-blind placebo-controlled study assessing impact of medical therapy on BPH progression (> 4 point rise in IPSS, development of AUR) (2003) [18]

3000+ men (mean prostate volume 36mL) randomized to one of four arms:
- placebo,
- doxazosin 8mg / day,
- finasteride 5mg / day,
- combination of doxazosin and finasteride, (mean follow-up of 4.5 years)

Found that combination therapy provided benefits over either drug as mono-therapy in terms of reduction in the risk of clinical progression.

CombAT (COMBination of Avodart and Tamsulosin) [19] (avodart = dutasteride)

4-yr, multi-centre, randomised, double-blind study (2008)

4800+ men aged ≥ 50 years with clinical diagnosis of BPH, IPSS > 12, randomised to:
- tamsulosin 400µg / day
- dutasteride 0.5mg / day
- combination of both

The findings of the study:
- combination superior to tamsulosin mono-therapy but not dutasteride monotherapy at reducing the relative risk of AUR or BPH-related surgery

- combination superior to both mono-therapies at reducing RR of BPH progression
- combination provided greater symptom benefit than either mono-therapy at 4 years

CONDUCT [20]

2 year multi-centre, randomised trial (2015)

700+ men, with treatment-naive BPH, IPSS (8–19) randomised to:
- combination of 0.5 mg dutasteride and 0.4 mg tamsulosin
- watchful waiting (WW)

The findings of the study:
- change in IPSS significantly greater for combination compared to WW
- risk of BPH progression reduced in combination group by 43%

PLESS (Proscar Long-Term Efficacy and Safety Study) [17] (proscar = finasteride)

Multi-centre, randomised, placebo-controlled trial (1998)

3000+ men randomized to receive finasteride or placebo for 4 years (the aim was to examine the long-term benefit of finasteride in men with symptomatic BPH)

The findings of the study:
- prostate volume in placebo (+ 14%) and finasteride (-18%)
- prostate volume in finasteride group reached nadir at 1 year and remained at this level
- symptom score and flow rate in finasteride group showed modest and progressive improvements, in contrast to placebo group, which were unchanged
- finasteride exhibited 57% reduction in risk of AUR and 55% of progression to surgery

Olmsted County Study [21]

Started in 1990s, random selection of > 2000 men to follow up their LUTS / risk of AUR / BOO surgery

- Demonstrated that BPH is age dependent and progressive, IPSS rises by 0.18 points / year, Q_{max} decreases 2% / year and risk of AUR increases with age

This study also identified risk factors for BPH progression and requirement of surgical treatment (detailed in "Acute urinary retention" below).

PHYTOTHERAPY

Alternative treatments for BPH are plant extracts (phytotherapy).

EAU Guidelines / NICE / AUA have not made recommendations on their use due to lack of efficacy trials.

Options include: saw palmetto, urtica dioica (stinging nettle), pygeum africanum.

TURP

TURP involves removing tissue from the transition zone of the prostate, whilst TUIncisionP involves incising the bladder outlet without tissue removal.

Bipolar-TURP has similar efficacy but lower peri-operative morbidity compared to monopolar.

Other groups of patients that may benefit from TURP (or HoLEP):
- recurrent AUR
- recurrent visible haematuria of prostatic origin refractory to 5α-RI therapy
- bladder stones
- high-pressure chronic retention of urine (HPCRU)
- recurrent UTIs due to BPH / PVR

EAU Guidelines (2019): [22]

- Offer TUIP to surgically treat moderate-to-severe LUTS in men with prostate size < 30mL, without a middle lobe (Level 1a)
- Offer bipolar- or monopolar TURP to surgically treat moderate-to-severe LUTS in men with prostate size of 30–80mL (Level 1a)

Efficacy

TURP confers 90% chance of symptom improvement in BPH causing BOO – voiding symptoms improve faster than storage symptoms.

Improvements include Q_{max} (+162%), IPSS (-70%) and PVR (-77%).

The upper limit for TURP is ≤ 80mL, above which HoLEP / open prostatectomy considered.

EAU Guidelines (2019): [22]

- Offer endoscopic enucleation of prostate or open prostatectomy to treat moderate-to-severe LUTS in men with prostate size > 80mL (Level 1a)

Side-Effects

Provide the appropriate BAUS information leaflet about TURP and discuss complications:

- early: transfusion (1%), sepsis (≤ 3%) and anaesthesia related
- late: urinary incontinence (rare), retrograde ejaculation (≤ 100%), ED (10%), stricture and re-do surgery (cumulative risk 2% / year, i.e. 10% at 5 years)

HOLEP

The holmium:yttrium-aluminium garnet (Ho:YAG) laser can be used to treat BOO.

Functions as solid-state laser absorbed by prostate tissue to a depth ≤ 0.4mm and the heat created (> 100°C) cause tissue vaporisation whilst coagulating blood vessels

The irrigation fluid is normal saline (avoids risk of TUR syndrome).

NICE Guidelines endorse use of HoLEP for larger prostates (> 80g), long-term efficacy is comparable to TURP.

Risks of ED and retrograde ejaculation comparable with TURP

Most common complication after HoLEP is dysuria, however compared to TURP it is associated with shorter catheterisation time and hospital stay.

UROLIFT™

Encroaching lateral lobes compressed by small permanent sutures under cystoscopic guidance, resulting in an opening of the prostatic urethra

It cannot be used to treat patients with large obstructing median lobe.

Urolift™ does not appear to have any impact on sexual / ejaculatory function.

EAU Guidelines (2019): [21]

- Offer prostatic urethral lift (Urolift™) to men with LUTS interested in preserving ejaculatory function, with prostates < 70mL and no middle lobe

ACUTE URINARY RETENTION

There are a number of risk factors for AUR. [Table 15]

Table 15 – risk factors for developing AUR

Risk Factor	AUR Relative Risk
IPSS > 7	3.2
Qmax < 12 mL/s	3.9
Prostate vol. > 30 mL	3.0
PSA > 1.4	2.0
Age > 70y vs. 40–49y	10–11
Unspecified volume of PVR	

Other risk factors include previous AUR and failure to respond to medical treatment.

The risk of AUR is 1% per year in patients with BPH.

High Pressure Chronic Retention of Urine (HPCRU)

HPCRU is an indication for catheterisation and subsequent BOO surgery.

Post-obstructive diuresis requires close monitoring of potassium, with an IV normal saline replacement of 2 / 3 the volume of previous hour's output.

Post-obstructive diuresis occurs physiologically due to accumulation of fluid / electrolyte in preceding period of renal failure.

Diuresis is defined as > 200mL / hour of urine output for 2 hours or more.

Pathological elements of diuresis include:
- poor response of collecting ducts to ADH
- increased production of ANP
- inability to maintain medullary solute gradient due to increased blood flow
- defective medullary solute gradient (reduced NaCL and urea reabsorption)

HPCRU develops gradually over time, as the bladder retains an ever-greater amount of urine after voiding (EVP – end void pressure).

The patient's bladder fills and the pressure rises until they void (EFP – end fill pressure) after which the pressure drops down to EVP again.

Only relief of the obstruction will bring the resting bladder pressure down. [Image 6]

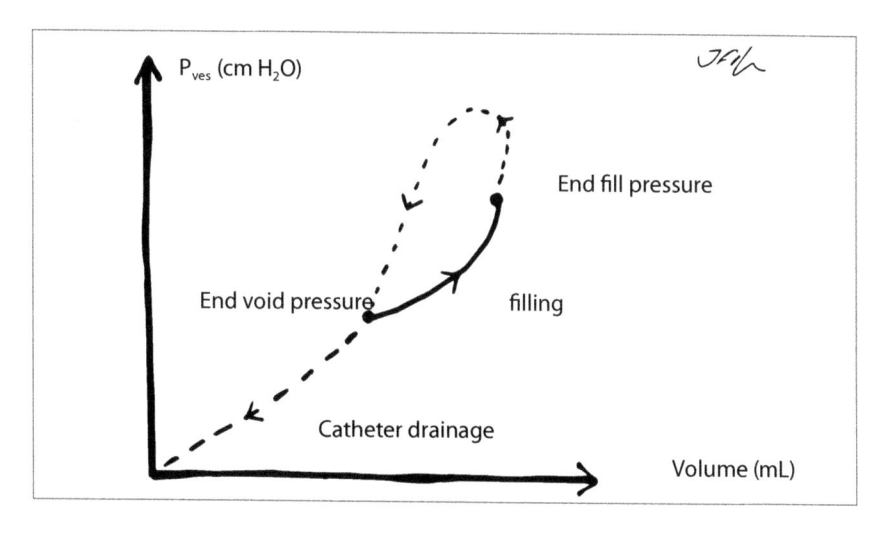

Image 6 – Graphical demonstration of bladder pressures in HPCRU

GFR takes ≤ 3 months to fully recover (plasma creatinine continues to decrease during period).

Recall that creatinine is excreted by tubules as well as through glomerular filtration, therefore tubular function recovers within 14 days but full glomerular function can take 3 months.

About 80% of creatinine clearance is due to GFR and 20% to renal tubular secretion.

Thus creatinine clearance is an over-estimate of actual GFR (ie. becomes important in renal failure where tubular secretion may be responsible for relatively greater proportion of clearance).

$99^{m}Tc$ DTPA (diethylene-triamine-penta-acetic acid) clearance another means of calculating GFR

NICE Recommendations on managing LUTS in men (2020) [23]

- Offer an α-1 blocker to men with moderate-to-severe LUTS
- Consider offering anti-cholinergic as well as α-1 blocker to men who still have storage symptoms after treatment with α-1 blocker alone
- Offer 5α-RI to men with LUTS with prostates > 30g and / or PSA > 1.4 ng / mL, and who are considered to be at high risk of progression
- Consider combination α-1 blocker and 5α-RI to men with bothersome moderate-to-severe LUTS and prostates > 30g and / or PSA > 1.4 ng / mL

VARICOCOELE

A varicocoele is abnormal dilatation of the veins in the pampiniform plexus of the spermatic cord.

The pampiniform plexus is formed from internal spermatic and gonadal veins.

EPIDEMIOLOGY

Estimated prevalence in 15% of men, however 25% of men with abnormal semen analysis

Rare prior to puberty

Varicocoele is left sided in 90% of cases.

AETIOLOGY

The fact that 90% of varicocoeles are left sided suggests reasons for its development:

- left testicular vein drains into left renal vein, higher pressure system
- absence of venous valves is more commonly found on the left side
- left renal vein may be compressed between SMA and aorta

There appears to be a correlation between varicocoele and infertility.

One theory relates to counter-current mechanism for heat exchange provided by pampiniform plexus to arteries entering testes, which is impaired by the varicocoele.

Semen analysis improvement is often noted after surgical correction of varicocoele (70%), particularly the sperm motility.

CLASSIFICATION

Varicocoeles are graded according to findings on physical examination. [Table 16]

Table 16 – grading of varicocoeles

Grade	Description
0	Sub-clinical (seen on USS only)
1	Palpable on valsalva manœuvre only
2	Palpable on standing, not visible
3	Palpable and visible

DIAGNOSTIC EVALUATION

The factors present in the *patient history* may include:
- heavy, dragging sensation in scrotum
- symptoms affected with position

In the presence of a chaperone the *patient examination* should assess for:
- palpable "bag of worms" in the scrotum
- repeat examination in lying and standing position
- assess ipsilateral testicular volume (often reduced)
- palpate ipsilateral kidney

The diagnostic examination of choice is *Scrotal Doppler US* (ensure to scan ipsilateral kidney).

MANAGEMENT

Improvement in semen parameters are seen in 70% of men undergoing surgical intervention.

Evers (2004) meta-analysis found varicocoele treatment did not improve pregnancy rates, however:
- Included patients with sub-clinical varicocoeles and normal semen parameters
- When these were excluded, 36% (treated) vs. 20% (untreated) [24]

Conservative

Many patients with varicocoeles do not require or wish to undergo treatment.

NICE does not recommend intervention on varicocoele purely in the context of infertility treatment as this does not improve pregnancy rates.

The following patients should be offered treatment:

- adolescents with Grade II / III varicocoele and reduced ipsilateral testicular volume
- sub-fertile males with impaired semen parameters (parameters are likely to improve, at least sufficient for IUI, IVF or ICSI)
- painful, symptomatic varicocoeles

Venous Embolisation

Interventional radiology embolisation is favoured as 1st line (coils or sclerosing agents).

Success rates > 80% are quoted

Patients must be counselled regarding recurrence after embolisation, delayed shrinkage of testicle and risk of sub-fertility.

Surgical Options

The spermatic / testicular vein can be clipped laparoscopically.

Open options include via inguinal (Ivanissevich) or high-retroperitoneal (Palomo) approaches.

REFERENCES

1. McNeal JE. (1981) The zonal anatomy of the prostate. *The prostate*, 2(1), 35–49.
2. Bartsch G, Rittmaster RS, Klocker H. (2000) Dihydrotestosterone and the concept of 5alpha-reductase inhibition in human benign prostatic hyperplasia. *European Urology*, 37 (4): 367–80.
3. Rittmaster R, Hahn RG, Ray P, et al. (2008). Effect of dutasteride on intraprostatic androgen levels in men with benign prostatic hyperplasia or prostate cancer. *Urology*, 72(4), 808–812.
4. Althof SE, McMahon CG, Waldinger MD, et al. (2014). An update of the International Society of Sexual Medicine's guidelines for the diagnosis and treatment of premature ejaculation (PE). *The journal of sexual medicine*, 11(6), 1392–1422.
5. https://www.baus.org.uk/_userfiles/pages/files/Patients/Leaflets/Vasectomy.pdf [Accessed 18 May 2020].
6. Grey BR, Thompson A, Jenkins BL, et al. (2012). UK practice regarding reversal of vasectomy 2001–2010: relevance to best contemporary patient management. *BJU international*, 110(7), 1040–1047.
7. Kalsi JS, Minhas S, Muneer A., Andrology. In: Arya M, Shergill I, Fernando HS et al. Viva Practice for the FRCS (Urol) and Postgraduate Urology Examinations 2nd Edition (2018) CRC Press, London.
8. National Institute for Health and Care Excellence (2017) Fertility problems" assessment and treatment [CG 156]. Available at: https://www.nice.org.uk/guidance/cg156 [last accessed 18 May 2020].
9. https://commons.wikimedia.org/wiki/File:Penis_cross_section.svg [last accessed 18 May 2020].
10. Rosen RC, Cappelleri JC, Smith MD, et al. (1999). Development and evaluation of an abridged, 5-item version of the International Index of Erectile Function (IIEF-5) as a diagnostic tool for erectile dysfunction. *International journal of impotence research*, 11(6), 319–326.
11. Gross MS, Phillips EA, Balen A, et al. (2016). The malleable implant salvage technique: infection outcomes after Mulcahy salvage procedure and replacement of infected inflatable penile prosthesis with malleable prosthesis. *The Journal of urology*, 195(3), 694–698.
12. Hackett G, Kirby M, Edwards D, et al. (2017). British Society for Sexual Medicine guidelines on adult testosterone deficiency, with statements for UK practice. *The journal of sexual medicine*, 14(12), 1504–1523.
13. Cooper TG, Noonan E, Von Eckardstein S, et al. (2010). World Health Organization reference values for human semen characteristics. *Human reproduction update*, 16(3), 231–245.

14. Hellstrom WJ, Feldman R, Rosen RC, et al. (2013). Bother and distress associated with Peyronie's disease: validation of the Peyronie's disease questionnaire. *The Journal of urology*, 190(2), 627–634.
15. Weidner W, Hauck EW, Schnitker J, et al. (2005). Potassium paraaminobenzoate (POTABA™) in the treatment of Peyronie's disease: a prospective, placebo-controlled, randomized study. *European urology*, 47(4), 530–536.
16. Barrett-Harlow B, Wang R, (2016). Oral therapy for Peyronie's disease, does it work?. *Translational andrology and urology*, 5(3), 296.
17. Roehrborn CG, Bruskewitz R, Nickel GC, et al. (2000). Urinary retention in patients with BPH treated with finasteride or placebo over 4 years. *European urology*, 37(5), 528–536.
18. McConnell JD, Roehrborn CG, Bautista OM, et al. (2003). The long-term effect of doxazosin, finasteride, and combination therapy on the clinical progression of benign prostatic hyperplasia. *New England Journal of Medicine*, 349(25), 2387–2398.
19. Roehrborn CG, Siami P, Barkin J. (2008) The effects of dutasteride, tamsulosin and combination therapy on lower urinary tract symptoms in men with benign prostatic hyperplasia and prostatic enlargement: 2-year results from the CombAT study. *The Journal of urology*, 179(2), 616–621.
20. Roehrborn CG, Oyarzabal Perez I, Roos EP. (2015) Efficacy and safety of a fixed-dose combination of dutasteride and tamsulosin treatment (D uodart®) compared with watchful waiting with initiation of tamsulosin therapy if symptoms do not improve, both provided with lifestyle advice, in the management of treatment-naïve men with moderately symptomatic benign prostatic hyperplasia: 2-year CONDUCT study results. *BJU international*, 116(3),450–459.
21. Jacobsen SJ, Jacobson DJ, Girman CJ, et al. (1999). Treatment for benign prostatic hyperplasia among community dwelling men: the Olmsted County study of urinary symptoms and health status. *The Journal of urology*, 162(4), 1301–1306.
22. Gravas S, Cornu JN, Gacci M, et al. (2019) EAU Guidelines on Management of Non-Neurogenic Male Lower Urinary Tract Symptoms (LUTS), incl. Benign Prostatic Obstruction (BPO). Available at: https://uroweb.org/wp-content/uploads/EAU-Guidelines-on-the-Management-of-Non-Neurogenic-Male-LUTS-2019.pdf [last accessed 19 May 2020].
23. NICE Pathway – lower urinary tract symptoms in men. Available at: https://pathways.nice.org.uk/pathways/lower-urinary-tract-symptoms-in-men [last accessed 19 May 2020].
24. Evers JL, Collins J, (2004) Surgery or embolisation for varicocele in subfertile men. *Cochrane Database of Systematic Reviews*, (3).

ANDROLOGY AND BPH MCQS

1. Which of the following statements is correct?
   A) Dutasteride inhibits type-1 5AR enzyme only
   B) Dutasteride inhibits both type-1 and type-2 5AR enzymes
   C) Finasteride inhibits type-1 5AR enzyme only
   D) Finasteride inhibits type-1 and type-2 5AR enzymes
   E) None of the above

2. Which medication can cause retrograde ejaculation as a side effect?
   A) Chloral hydrate
   B) Chlorambucil
   C) Chlordiazepoxide
   D) Chlorpromazine
   E) None of the above

3. Testosterone supplementation may cause one of the following:
   A) Basophilia
   B) Eosinophilia
   C) Rise in haematocrit
   D) Thrombocytopenia
   E) None of the above

4. Which of the following statements is correct?
   A) LH decreases cholesterol desmolase activity
   B) Prolactin decreases the response of Leydig cells to LH
   C) Leydig cells are polyhedral in shape
   D) Testosterone provides positive feedback to the hypothalamus
   E) None of the above

5. Which of the following statements regarding Peyronie's disease is incorrect?
   A) It is more common in Caucasian rather than Afro-Caribbean men
   B) Typical age of onset is 60–70 years
   C) Penile ultrasonography typically reveals hyperechoic thickened tunica albuginea
   D) It is associated with Ledderhose disease
   E) Tamoxifen modulates fibroblast secretion and thus more effective in acute phase

6. Which of the following is not a recognised side effect of tamsulosin?
   A) Papillitis
   B) Asthenia
   C) Stevens-Johnson syndrome
   D) Angioedema
   E) Diarrhoea

7. Which of the following is not a recognised risk factor for developing AUR?
   A) IPSS > 5
   B) PSA > 1.4
   C) $Q_{max} < 12mL/s$
   D) Age > 70 years
   E) Prostate volume > 30mL

8. Which phytotherapy agent has not been used to treat BPH symptoms?
   A) Pygeum africanum
   B) Saw palmetto
   C) Beta-sitosterol
   D) Secale cereale
   E) Ferula persica

9. Regarding surgical treatment for Peyronie's disease, which of the following statements is true?
   A) The most commonly used autograft for the Lue procedure is the saphenous vein
   B) Lue procedure has a lower risk of ED than Nesbit plication
   C) Yachia procedure is a form of concave lengthening procedure
   D) 75% of patients undergoing Nesbit's procedure will require a circumcision
   E) Residual penile curvature < 20° after plication is uncommon in high-volume centres

10. An isolated deficiency in LH is found in which condition?
    A) Kallman syndrome
    B) Leydig cell hypoplasia
    C) Swyer syndrome
    D) Pasqualini syndrome
    E) Jacob's syndrome

STATION 8: BPH AND ANDROLOGY

11. Which one of the following lower reference limit values as per WHO (2010) semen analysis parameters is incorrect?

    A) Sperm morphology > 4% normal forms
    B) Total sperm count > 39 x 10^6
    C) Sperm concentration > 12 x 10^6 / mL
    D) Semen volume > 1.5 mL
    E) Progressive motility > 32%

12. Which of the following is not a symptom that features on the IPSS questionnaire?

    A) Straining
    B) Intermittency
    C) Urgency
    D) Incomplete emptying
    E) Hesitancy

13. Which of the following is not a recognised side effect of sildenafil?

    A) Gynaecomastia
    B) Oculogyric crisis
    C) Myalgia
    D) Insomnia
    E) Scleral discoloration

14. What approximate proportion of patients treated with PDE5i drugs do not respond?

    A) 5%
    B) 10%
    C) 20%
    D) 30%
    E) 40%

15. The CONDUCT study for BPH evaluated the following medication against watchful waiting:

    A) Dutasteride and alfuzosin
    B) Dutasteride and terazosin
    C) Finasteride and alfuzosin
    D) Finasteride and terazosin
    E) None of the above

16. Which artery does the common penile artery arise from?
    A) Internal pudendal artery
    B) Anterior branch of internal iliac artery
    C) Posterior branch of internal iliac artery
    D) External pudendal artery
    E) Superficial external pudendal artery

17. Where is the somatic centre for efferent innervation of ischio- and bulbo-cavernous muscles of the penis?
    A) Onuf's nucleus
    B) Marginal nucleus
    C) Nucleus propius
    D) Nucleus solitarius
    E) Edinger-Westphal nucleus

18. What proportion of circulating testosterone is free?
    A) < 1%
    B) 2%
    C) 5%
    D) 10%
    E) 20%

19. The precursor to the primary spermatocyte is:
    A) preleptotene spermatocyte
    B) Intermediate spermatogonium
    C) spermatid
    D) type-A spermatogonium
    E) type-B spermatogonium

20. Globozoospermia is best defined as:
    A) increase in viscosity of sperm
    B) high percentage of immotile sperm
    C) sperm lacking acrosomal caps
    D) high percentage of dead sperm
    E) sperm heads are tapered

21. The mechanism of action of POTABA to treat Peyronie's disease is best described as:
    A) inhibits collagen by increasing serotonin levels
    B) activates free radicals to reduce oxidative stress
    C) Inactivates free radicals to reduce oxidative stress
    D) Increases serotonin levels to decrease fibrosis
    E) Decreases serotonin levels to decrease fibrosis

22. What is the average half-life of unbound testosterone?
    A) 24–48 hours
    B) ≤ 24 hours
    C) ≤ 6 hours
    D) 10–15 minutes
    E) < 5 minutes

23. Which of the following statements regarding Urolift™ is true?
    A) MRI is safe provided the static magnetic field is of ≤ 3 Tesla
    B) MRI is safe provided the static magnetic field is of ≤ 5 Tesla
    C) Patients with Urolift™ should not have an MRI scan
    D) It is safe in all MRI scanners
    E) None of the above

24. Which of the following criteria does not feature on the IIEF-5 questionnaire for ED?
    A) Patient difficulty in maintaining an erection after penetration
    B) Patient frequency of achieving erection adequate for penetration
    C) Patient difficulty in maintaining an erection to complete intercourse
    D) Patient perceived rigidity of erection
    E) Patient frequency of satisfaction in sexual intercourse

25. What is the half-life of tadalafil?
    A) ~ 24 hours
    B) ~ 17 hours
    C) ~ 13 hours
    D) ~ 9 hours
    E) ~ 6 hours

26. Which of the following statements regarding Doppler study of penile blood flow in erection for EDC assessment is true?
    A) End diastolic velocity is normal if > 10 cm / s
    B) End diastolic velocity is normal if > 5 cm / s
    C) Peak systolic velocity is abnormal if < 25 cm / s
    D) Peak systolic velocity is abnormal if < 35 cm / s
    E) None of the above

27. Which of the following groups of IIEF-5 questionnaire scores is correct as per the different categories of ED severity?
    A) 1–6, 7–10, 11–15, 16–21, 22–25
    B) 1–7, 8–11, 12–16, 17–21, 22–25
    C) 1–5, 6–10, 11–16, 17–21, 22–25
    D) 1–7, 8–12, 13–17, 18–21, 22–25
    E) 1–6, 7–10, 11–15, 16–20, 21–25

28. What is the correct late failure rate for vasectomy?
    A) 1 in 500
    B) 1 in 1000
    C) 1 in 1500
    D) 1 in 2000
    E) 1 in 2500

29. All of the following are contra-indications to PDE5i use except:
    A) Active peptic ulceration
    B) Hereditary degenerative retinal disorder
    C) History of non-arteritic anterior ischaemic optic neuropathy
    D) Recent history of antero-lateral myocardial infarction
    E) Recent history of postero-lateral myocardial infarction

30. Which of the following statements about PDE5i drugs is true?
    A) they convert ATP to cAMP
    B) they convert GTP to GMP
    C) they convert GMP to cGMP
    D) they convert GTP to cGMP
    E) they convert cGMP to GMP

ANSWERS TO MCQS

STATION 5: CALCULI AND URINARY TRACT INFECTIONS
1. **B** – low calcium intake is correct
2. **D**
3. **A**
4. **A**
5. **C**
6. **B** – cysteine should be "cystine" (cystine is oxidised dimer form of cysteine)
7. **C**
8. **A**
9. **E**
10. **E** – bulinus is the intermediate snail host for S.haematobium, not S.mansoni (the name of the intermediate host is biomphalaria)
11. **D** – isoniazid may cause peripheral neuropathy
12. **C**
13. **B**
14. **A** – weddelite is calcium oxalate dihydrate
15. **A**
16. **D** – renal leak hypercalciuria is associated with medullary sponge kidney
17. **D** – acetohydraamic acid is a competitive inhibitor of urease (its molecule is similar to urea but not hydrolysable by urease), pH ≥ 7.2 favours staghorn formation
18. **E** – nitrofurantoin is potentially harmful in pregnancy as may cause haemolytic anaemia
19. **C** – penicillamine binds to cysteine
20. **B**
21. **B**
22. **A** – mumps is an RNA paramyxovirus disease
23. **D**
24. **C**
25. **E** – chlamydia is a gram-negative coccus, but it is also an obligate parasite (i.e. cannot complete life cycle without host exploitation) (holoparasite is another term for obligate parasite)

STATION 6: UROLOGICAL IMAGING & PRINCIPLES OF UROLOGICAL TECHNOLOGY

1. **D** – polypropylene is prolene, which is non-absorbable
2. **A**
3. **B**
4. **C**
5. **A**
6. **E**
7. **E**
8. **B**
9. **D** – recall the diameter corresponds to a 1/3 of the French gauge.
10. **C**
11. **A**
12. **C**
13. **D**
14. **B**
15. **E**
16. **C**
17. **A**
18. **B**
19. **B**
20. **E**

STATION 7: BLADDER DYSFUNCTION AND GYNAECOLOGICAL ASPECTS OF UROLOGY

1. **C**
2. **B**
3. **E**
4. **A** – heart failure is a caution, not a contraindication
5. **E**
6. **C**
7. **E**
8. **D** – note the doses given were 200units and 300units (neuropaths are usually offered a higher starting dose compared to patients with IDO)
9. **E**
10. **D** – in this case duloxetine should be stopped, however it is recommended always to taper down the dose over 1–2 weeks
11. **C**
12. **A**
13. **B**

14. B
15. C
16. D
17. D – the intrinsic sphincter is absent posteriorly
18. A
19. E – angioedema is rare, it is metabolised by the liver but indeed excreted in the urine
20. B

STATION 8: ANDROLOGY AND BPH

1. B
2. D – chlorpromazine is an anti-psychotic drug which also possesses anti-serotonergic properties.
3. C – the haematocrit should be checked at baseline and yearly if testosterone treatment ongoing
4. C
5. B – Peyronie's is most common in men 50–60 years
6. A
7. A – IPSS > 7 is a recognised risk factor for developing AUR in men
8. E
9. A – note that circumcision required in 25%, and minor residual curvature is common
10. D
11. C – sperm concentration > 15×10^6 / mL (WHO semen analysis parameters are an exam favourite, and these should be memorised confidently
12. E
13. B
14. D
15. E – CONDUCT study evaluated dutasteride and tamsulosin, it is essential for the BPH station to have learned an overview of each of the major BPH trials (e.g. MTOPS, PLESS, COMBAT)
16. A
17. A
18. B
19. E
20. C
21. E
22. D
23. A

24. D
25. B
26. C
27. B
28. D
29. A – sildenafil can be prescribed with caution in peptic ulcer disease
30. E

Milton Keynes UK
Ingram Content Group UK Ltd.
UKHW021821290924
448966UK00009B/96